Detox Your Place

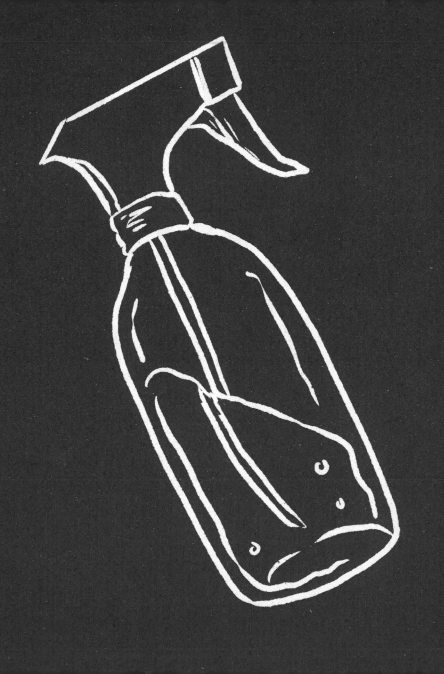

Detox Your Place

Room by Room Remedies for Nontoxic Living

Meadow Shadowhawk

Microcosm Publishing
Portland, OR

DETOX YOUR PLACE
Room by Room Remedies for Nontoxic Living
Part of the DIY Series

© Meadow Shadowhawk, 2020
This edition © Microcosm Publishing, 2020
First Edition, 3,000 copies, first published August, 2020

ISBN 978-1-62106-149-6
This is Microcosm #312
Designed by Joe Biel
Edited by Sarah Koch

For a catalog, write or visit:
Microcosm Publishing
2752 N Williams Ave.
Portland, OR 97227
(503)799-2698
MicrocosmPublishing.com

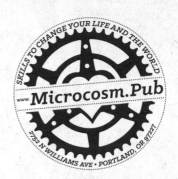

If you bought this on Amazon, I'm so sorry because you could have gotten it cheaper and supported a small, independent publisher at www.Microcosm.Pub

To join the ranks of high-class stores that feature Microcosm titles, talk to your local rep: In the U.S. **Como** (Atlantic), **Fujii** (Midwest), **Book Travelers West** (Pacific), **Turnaround** in Europe, **UTP/Manda** in Canada, **New South** in Australia, and **GPS** in Asia, Africa, India, South America, and other countries. We are sold in the gift market by **Gifts of Nature.**

Global labor conditions are bad, and our roots in industrial Cleveland in the 70s and 80s made us appreciate the need to treat workers right. Therefore, our books are MADE IN THE USA and printed on post-consumer paper.

Library of Congress Cataloging-in-Publication Data
Names: Shadowhawk, Meadow, author.
Title: Detox your place : room-by-room remedies for nontoxic living / by Meadow Shadowhawk.
Description: Portland, OR : Microcosm Publishing, 2020. | Includes
    bibliographical references. | Summary: "Looking to detox your home without the use of harsh
    chemicals, overly processed cleaning products, or by any other questionable means? Meadow
    Shadowhawk will help you through the process, with well-researched advice about topics like
    making your own cleaning products, selecting paint, choosing a vacuum cleaner, and even
    replacing furniture and insulation. Includes recipes for creating your own versions of everyday
    items, tips on what to buy (and what to avoid!), and what the facts are about various things. This
    book is a guide to overhauling your home to make it safer and more comfortable for yourself,
    your family, and your pets. Here's to living a happier, healthier life!"-- Provided by publisher.
Identifiers: LCCN 2019058701 (print) | LCCN 2019058702 (ebook) | ISBN
    9781621061496 | ISBN 9781621061953 (ebook)
Subjects: LCSH: House cleaning. | Household supplies. | Housing and health.
    | Natural products.
Classification: LCC TX324 .S435 2020 (print) | LCC TX324 (ebook) | DDC
    648/.5--dc23
LC record available at https://lccn.loc.gov/2019058701
LC ebook record available at https://lccn.loc.gov/2019058702

MICROCOSM · PUBLISHING

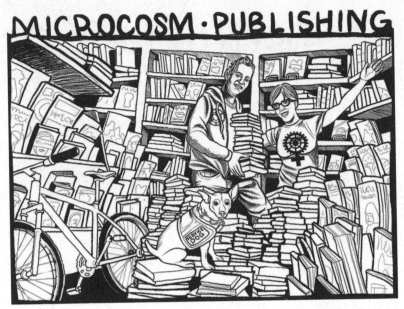

Microcosm Publishing is Portland's most diversified publishing house and distributor with a focus on the colorful, authentic, and empowering. Our books and zines have put your power in your hands since 1996, equipping readers to make positive changes in your life and in the world around you. Microcosm emphasizes skill-building, showing hidden histories, and fostering creativity through challenging conventional publishing wisdom. What was once a distro and record label was started by Joe Biel in his bedroom and has become among the oldest independent publishing houses in Portland, OR. In a world that has inched to the right for 80 years, we are carving out a place in the center with DIY skills, food, bicycling, gender, self-care, and social justice.

Table of Contents

Introduction

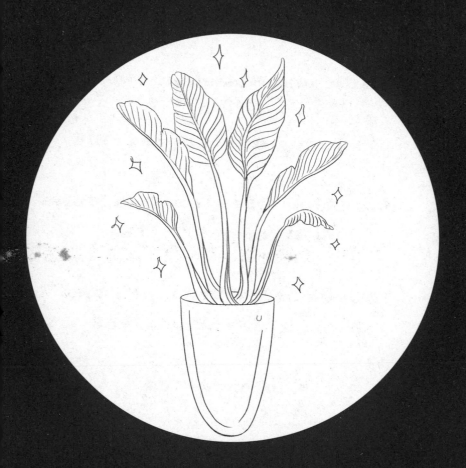

*A*s a mother of two living in a world where we have managed to compromise our air, land, water, and food, I am keenly aware not only of how things affect me and my family but also future generations. Our everyday actions not only affect us, but have a ripple effect that extends to our family, our community, and eventually, to the entire world. The future our descendants will inherit is dependent on the actions we take in the present.

Just as we are living with polluted air, toxic water supplies, and less nutritious food sources handed down to us by our parents, we must consider what we will leave for our children. Most Native Americans have long had a philosophy of basing their decisions on how their actions will affect the next seven generations. Having Native American heritage, I have always been guided by this principle and I am confident that if the world's governments had this same philosophy, our world would look quite different. As humans progress, we are becoming more and more technologically advanced, but in regards to the overall health of mankind and the planet, we are decelerating at an alarming rate.

When working as a veterinarian technician in the early 1980s, I learned about a pet food developer who created a "natural" product, free of artificial colors or additives. He did this because research had shown a possible connection between these additives and birth defects as well as other illnesses. Having learned this, he sought to provide an alternative for those that wanted to avoid them in their pet food. That was a wakeup call for me. Like many people, I always thought that if something was allowed in the food supply, it must be safe. However, coming to the realization that that may not always be the case is what kick started my own research, a task which has been made all the more complicated in our current age of mega corporations doing whatever they can to increase profits. For the past twenty years, industrial facilities have continued to encroach on my suburban neighborhood. In that time, we have witnessed an alarming number of friends and neighbors diagnosed with various cancers, fibromyalgia, chronic migraines, asthma, and allergies, to name just a few ailments. Adding to this the number of local pets that have died from mysterious kidney diseases or succumbed to cancer at a young age, I began to wonder if it had to do with the environment we lived in.

Unfortunately it is not only my suburban neighborhood, city, state, or even country that is affected. Many people today are dealing with the effects of toxic environments, medical treatments, or just everyday life in a world that puts monetary gains before the health interests of its inhabitants. Most people are not even aware of the myriad of toxins that surround them, or what they can do about them. As regulations protecting people from harmful elements are eliminated or reduced in an effort to stimulate the economy, we are increasing the danger to people, the environment, and even the world.

It is therefore my intention in this book to provide you with the information needed to identify potentially harmful elements in your home, and explain how to replace them with nontoxic alternatives. Organized by rooms and subjects, this is the result of decades of research collected, scrutinized, and practiced in an effort to survive in our ever deteriorating world.

Things are constantly changing, and in the name of progress and convenience we have developed a lifestyle filled with toxic substances. Keeping up with the latest information on any given product can be time consuming and downright overwhelming. One day CFL light bulbs are the best bulbs to save the environment, and the next year we find out they emit high levels of ultraviolet radiation—specifically UVC and UVA rays.[1] Experts say this radiation could initiate cell death and even cause skin cancer.[2] So maybe LED lights would be better? Well, now we have learned that some LED lights are bad for the environment due to their high lead and arsenic content, and are bad for your health, mood, and can promote blindness, as the blue lights could possibly lead to age-related macular degeneration.[3] It turns out that the best lighting for your health and happiness may actually just be the good old fashioned incandescent light bulbs.

While detoxification may seem overwhelming and you may feel hopeless, you do have an element of control. By being aware of what may be toxic, and how to substitute nontoxic alternatives, you can more easily maintain a healthy lifestyle. Most of the solutions are very cost effective and not labor intensive. Those that are more labor intensive can be done with some elbow-grease or will come with store-bought suggestions.

It is important to remember that whatever toxins can affect you, they are even more detrimental to your children and your pets.

When you do make changes, it may be a good idea to do it in steps rather than all at once. Sometimes if we try to do too much at one time it can be overwhelming and cause you to give up all together. Small steps are progress and will lead to success when they are continued. To make this a bit easier, the book is arranged by rooms. It will point out potential problems and provide solutions. Even if you are unable to make all of the changes suggested, doing whatever you can will lessen the toxic load in your home. This is only a guide to build on, to help you get started with the things you do have control over in order to live a less toxic life.

Living Room

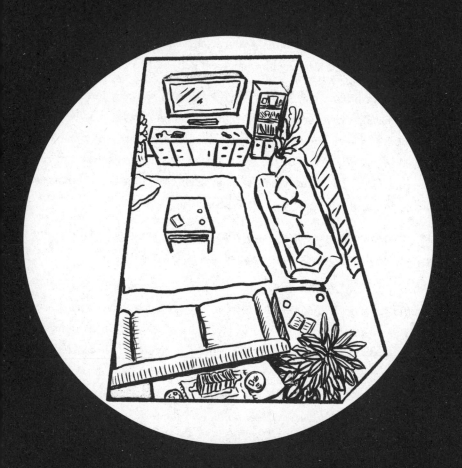

*T*he living room is most likely the first space you encounter as you enter a home. It is a gathering place where family and friends spend hours, children and pets spend much of their day playing on the floor, and it is often the focal point of the household. It is not typically one you would think would have many toxic risks. However, you might be surprised.

Toxins in this room can come from anything from carpeting, vinyl floor covering, paints and varnishes, or even from the flame retardants in the foam and cloth of your furniture. These generally include, but are not limited to: TDCPP, listed as a carcinogen by the state of California in 2011; PentaBDE, globally banned due to toxicity and environmental persistence; and Firemaster 550, which pilot studies have linked, even at low level exposures, to heart defects, obesity, and anxiety in animals.[4] Measurable concentrations of these toxins can be found in household dust and in thin films coating windows and surfaces. In fact, indoor air pollution can be up to five times higher than the air outside.[5]

If you can afford to purchase the less toxic alternatives such as VOC-free paint, flame retardant-free furniture with petroleum free foam, using solid wood frames, certified organic textiles, and water based adhesives, then you are in good shape. If you are like most of us however, and are not in this position, then you need to do what you can to lessen the toxic load.

Some of the simplest things like opening your windows for five to ten minutes a day to allow fresh air to flush out any concentrations of chemicals, or removing your shoes when you enter to avoid bringing in whatever toxic chemicals you may have walked through can make a big difference. Little changes can have a big impact. Just adding a few of the right plants can even improve the air quality in your home.

Air Fresheners and Potpourri

Scent is one of our strongest senses. Not only does our olfactory system identify smells, it influences taste and acts as a huge trigger for bringing up memories. For some, the smell of a pine tree in winter conjures up happy memories of the holidays. The smell of freshly baked bread or a good marinara sauce on the stove is always inviting; even just a clean fresh scent can be appealing. Our strong relation to scent is why there is an entire industry dedicated to providing products that attract our noses. The problem here is that the air fresheners promising these wonderful memory-making scents are full of chemicals that can accumulate in the human body, causing fatigue, migraines, asthma, allergies, and cancer, among other ailments. Studies of air fresheners revealed high levels of phthalates, hormone-disrupting chemicals that can be particularly dangerous for young children and unborn babies.[6] Air fresheners and cleaning products do not have to go through safety testing processes before being sold in stores because they are self-regulated by the cleaning industry.[7] It is no surprise then, that products labeled "all natural" and "unscented" were found to contain phthalates that were not disclosed in the list of ingredients.[8] Synthetic fragrances are another problem entirely. A large number of them are made from petroleum and cause issues ranging from asthma and allergies to changes in blood pressure and migraines.[9]

All of these chemicals, of which there are more than 350 to choose from, can accumulate in the fatty tissues of one's body and build up over time. This makes losing weight more difficult since the body has a harder time breaking down the fat and releasing stored toxins back into the body.[10] Some air fresheners even contain the chemical 1,4-Dichlorobenzene, which has been shown to have adverse health effects on the nervous system and can temporarily block your sense of smell.[11]

The Alternatives:

Essential oils: Quality essential oils can be used in a variety of ways to not only make your home smell wonderful but even to improve the quality of the air. It is important to note that not all essential oils are equal. Some may be altered by adding synthetic chemicals or are sometimes diluted with vegetable oil (more information on essential oils is available in the chapter on Shopping for Alternatives). Placing a few drops of essential oil on the air intake filter of your vacuum cleaner before you use it makes the whole house smell like whatever fragrance you have chosen. Lavender essential oil is said to produce a calming atmosphere. Orange essential oil is a fresh scent currently being studied for stress reduction and is showing great promise in helping to minimize the symptoms of Post Traumatic Stress Disorder.[12] Lemongrass essential oil is known for its ability to repel insects, such as mosquitoes and ants, and its citrus scent helps relieve stress, anxiety, irritability, insomnia, and prevent drowsiness.[13] Maybe add a nice pine essential oil scent during the holidays to make the whole house smell festive.

Those of us who are old enough can remember the days when, if you had a cold, Vicks VapoRub was placed in the vaporizer to help you breathe easier, but while it worked by releasing eucalyptus scent into the air, it was also an extreme fire hazard. If someone in your home is suffering from a cold or congestion, simply use some eucalyptus oil to help clear things up for them instead. In addition to adding a few drops of whatever oil you choose to the vacuum filter, it can also be added to the furnace filter in the winter or air conditioning filter in the summer. However, it is important to make sure that the oil is not flammable when using it around the furnace intake. Even putting a few drops on a cotton pad and clipping it to a small fan will fill the room with a safe, nontoxic fragrance. If you are interested in providing a more constant scent you can use an essential oil diffuser. Nebulizers or ultrasonic diffusers work well, and there is even an effective heat diffuser suitable for use in the car.

You should avoid using essential oils in diffusers if you have pets or small children as they can be harmful to those with sensitive respiratory systems or just generally toxic to them. Always keep essential oils well out of reach of any pets or small children, as ingestion is extremely harmful.

Zeolite rocks: Zeolite is a natural mineral formed by volcanic ash over millions of years that absorbs odors, and even moisture in the air. Zeolite is so effective at absorbing bacterial odors and toxins that it was used to clean up the nuclear accidents at Chernobyl and Three Mile Island.[14] Zeolite rocks are readily available and usually sold in open weave bags that can be placed in the offending area. These rocks can be used in many ways:

- They help fruit last longer when placed in the bottom of the bowl.

- They keep your kitchen garbage pail from smelling when placed near the plastic lining,

- They help remove cigarette smell from carpeting and upholstery when left in a decorative bowl in the living room, and

- Placing a bag of rocks near your dog's bed or cat litter box will help to control animal odors (Zeolite rocks are nontoxic to animals).

- Place a bag of rocks under the seat in your car to keep it smelling fresh.

The great thing about these rocks is that they can be recharged over and over again by placing the bag in the sun for an afternoon. Or if that is not an option you can simply put the bag of rocks in a 200-degree oven for about an hour. Either way they will be ready for use again. Note: Zeolite rocks can create a powdery dust when shaken, it is always a good idea to avoid breathing dust from any source.

Candles

Candles are used to set a relaxing atmosphere, however, like air fresheners they too can be a source of toxic chemicals in your home. Generally, you'll want to avoid scented candles and other mass-produced ones. Making your own at home with wax from a source you trust is a great way to avoid all of these issues. Scented and dyed candles release chemicals when burned, as well as having lead or lead cores in the wick that can release dangerous amounts of lead and soot into your home.[15] Two very toxic chemicals, benzene and toluene, are found in the sooty residue from burning candles. Benzene has been identified as a carcinogen and, in large doses, toluene adversely affects the central nervous system. Some people are so sensitive to scented candles that they can trigger an asthma attack or migraines even if the candles are not being burned. Making your own at home, with wax from a source you trust, is a great way to avoid these issues.[16]

The Alternatives: *Beeswax candles:* Pure beeswax candles are available in un-dyed styles or made with nontoxic dyes. When purchasing beeswax candles it is important to check the label to ensure they are 100% beeswax. Some companies will label their product as beeswax candles even though they contain only a small portion of beeswax combined with regular paraffin.

Soy candles: Pure soy candles burn clean, emit no harmful fumes, and have very long burn times as well. As mentioned above it is important to read the label to be sure you are getting what you pay for. Look for 100% soy and natural scents and dyes as the only things listed. If it lists the word fragrance on the label it may be from a synthetic source and should be avoided.

Carpeting

More than half of the homes in America have carpeting, and whether old or new, carpets can contain a whole host of toxic chemicals. These include toluene, benzene, formaldehyde, ethyl benzene, styrene, and acetone all of which have made the EPA's list of Extremely Hazardous Substances.[17] Adhesives, foam padding, stain protectors, mothproofing, and flame retardants are all culprits in the toxic carpet stew. Old carpets are no better as they may contain chemicals that have been banned in recent years as well as holding up to eight times their weight in dust mites, dirt, pesticides, and other toxins brought in on shoes, feet, and paws.[18] So, what can you do? Well you can remove the carpeting from your home, as many people who suffer from allergies have done, or you can take steps to minimize the effects of having carpeting. A good doormat at the entry, removing your shoes, and using a high quality sealed HEPA (high efficiency particulate air) vacuum cleaner are all steps in the right direction. Open your windows often to ventilate your home, and consider a HEPA air filter for your home. If you do want carpeting, you should look for one made of naturally flame-retardant fibers such as wool or hemp. Hemp rugs are more resistant to mold and mildew than wool and can be used in rooms where moisture is an issue, like a bathroom or kitchen. You can also find beautiful natural carpeting made from plant fibers such as corn leaves and stalks, seagrass, jute, and coconut-husk fiber. Another advantage of natural fiber carpets is that, when they have served their usefulness and are no longer needed, they can be composted rather than added to the toxic load headed to the landfills. If you are looking to purchase carpeting, keep an eye out for the Green Label Plus certification, as it indicates the lowest-emitting carpet, adhesive, and cushion products on the market. However, the Green Label Plus program is run by the Carpet and Rug industry, so ask for the manufacturer's certification on environmental claims. Also be careful of "recycled" carpets, which are made from recycled materials and can include byproducts from coal-fired power plants that may contain toxic heavy metals. Once you have found your carpet, attach it with staples rather than gluing it to the floor. When you are having your carpet installed, have it unrolled and allow it to air-out in a well-ventilated space for 72 hours prior to installation.

Carpet cleaners: Clean, fresh carpets are part of having a clean house. When they look and smell nice, they give the impression that they are fine to spend time exercising or playing on with the kids. However, depending on how the carpets are cleaned that may or may not be true. Carpets act as a filter in your home to trap dust and dirt that might otherwise end up in the air. Young children and pets spend a lot of their time on the carpets, so it is important to make sure that it is a safe environment for them. Even the household cleaning products used to clean stains from your rug can leave a residue that will be absorbed, inhaled, or picked up by an animal. Most professional carpet cleaners use toxic chemicals like perchloroethylene and naphthalene, and while they are great at dissolving the dirt in your carpet, they can be dangerous to the human central nervous system and are potentially carcinogenic.[19] These professionals will often recommend using a stain resistant on your carpet after they clean it but these too can be loaded with toxic chemicals and should be avoided. Some professional carpet cleaners are using a method that uses oxygenated water, a nontoxic, effective, and safe alternative. When doing it yourself, a steam cleaner is a good way to combat stains and even small areas of carpeting using only hot water.

The Alternatives: To keep your carpets fresh and flea free:

- 1 part **Borax** (I use ¼ cup)

- 2 parts **Baking soda** (I use ½ cup)

- A few drops of **Essential oil** (optional)

The amount you choose to use of each will depend on how large an area you are treating. This recipe will be sufficient for a 10'x 12' area, depending on the saturation.

Place in a container with a shaker top or punch holes in the lid.

Shake the contents well to mix thoroughly, then sprinkle over the entire carpet. This can be left on the carpets overnight if you prefer or for a minimum of half an hour to absorb odors.

Vacuum carpets thoroughly.

The borax helps to clean and disinfect, the baking soda deodorizes, and any residue left behind in the carpet after vacuuming deters flea infestation. Borax is completely natural. It doesn't cause cancer, accumulate in the body, or absorb through the skin, and it is not harmful to the environment. Even leaving it for only an hour is fine and walking around on it only helps to work it into the carpet fibers. That being said, I would vacuum it up before allowing babies to crawl around on it or pets to sleep on it, particularly if you use essential oils in the mix.

For light stain removal:

- 1 part **white vinegar**

- 1 part **water**

Mix and spray onto the stain and allow it to sit for a few minutes.

Blot with a cloth.

For more stubborn stains, try diluted **castile soap** and **warm water** sprayed on the area and lightly scrubbed with a toothbrush, blot with cloth then rinse until clean.

Furniture

Because of flammability laws, most furniture and baby products contain flame retardants in the foam and cloth, and in chemically treated wood. These chemicals continuously migrate out of products into household dust, and are ingested or inhaled by humans and pets. Babies are further exposed through their mother's milk and household dust, which they ingest at higher levels due to their hand-to-mouth behavior.[20] These chemicals have been linked to everything from lower IQ's to cancer.[21]

Flame retardants: Some of these highly toxic flame retardants were banned in the U.S. in 2004, so only furniture made prior to that would contain those particular chemicals. But the Federal Chemical Safety Act allows those that were banned to be substituted by other potentially problematic chemicals. The manufacturers of consumer products are not required to disclose the results of toxicity tests to the public before selling their products.[22] To make matters worse as a consumer there is no way to know what the furniture you are buying is treated with because the United States does not require labeling on furniture contents beyond fiber types and quantities. A journalist with the Chicago Tribune's investigation revealed that an organization known as Citizens for Fire Safety, mounted a campaign to increase the use of fire-retardant chemicals in household furniture, electronics, baby products, and other goods. The group also sponsored witnesses who testified before state legislators in favor of flame retardants. The problem with this organization was that they were made up of the three largest makers of flame retardants in the world. The campaign worked and flame retardants are used in nearly everything in your living room (as well as other parts of your house) from carpeting to the plastic surrounding your television set.[23]

It can make you feel like the deck is stacked against you. So, what can you look for in safe non toxic furniture for you and your family? You really have to investigate the furniture you are considering buying. Just because a product is labeled with "eco-friendly" or "green" doesn't necessarily mean it is nontoxic. You may find something with flame retardant free organic cotton fabric, but the foam inside could be petroleum based and the wood frame may be particle board containing formaldehyde. Unfortunately, truly nontoxic furniture tends to be very expensive and limited in color but there are companies committed to providing such products. EcoBalanza, Pacific Rim Natural Maple Bedroom Furniture, and Carolina Morning are examples of companies making an effort to provide nontoxic furniture.   It is still important to question everything that goes into the piece you are looking at. Ask to see the fact sheets or any information the manufacturer can provide to certify their claims. Another safe alternative can be antique furniture; it is typically made of solid wood frames and is usually flame retardant free. If you are interested in having your current furniture tested, Duke University has you covered. Through a project funded by the National Institute of Environmental Health Sciences (NIEHS), any US resident can submit a sample of polyurethane foam (PUF) from their furniture, infant car seat, or any other product containing PUF. They will test for seven common flame retardant chemicals and mail back a report with the findings in about eight weeks.[24]

Furniture polish: The most common ingredient in conventional furniture polish, nitrobenzene, can cause skin and eye infections, respiratory tract irritations, and can be absorbed through your skin. Aerosol furniture polish has microscopic particles which contain carcinogenic chemicals that can end up in the bloodstream. Formaldehyde is a common ingredient found in these products, which is a known carcinogen that can accumulate in human fat tissue over time. Complete ingredients are not always shown, and if they are, they can be hard to understand. However, if you read the warnings on the label you'll see they can cause skin irritation, vision loss, or a trip to the emergency room if accidentally swallowed. If that weren't enough, it can cause severe damage to your lungs if inhaled.[25]

The Alternatives:

Furniture polish for wood:

- 1 cup **extra virgin olive oil**
- ½ cup **lemon juice**

Mix extra virgin olive oil with the lemon juice, shake well in a glass container. Apply a small amount to furniture with a soft cloth.

- 1 tsp **jojoba oil**
- ½ cup **white vinegar**

Mix the jojoba oil with half a cup of white vinegar and apply with a soft cloth. Enjoy clean and shining furniture without the toxic chemicals.

For restoring furniture:

- ½ cup **flaxseed oil**
- ½ cup **white vinegar**
- 2 tbsp fresh **lemon juice**

Mix flaxseed oil with white vinegar and add fresh lemon juice.

Shake well in a glass container and apply a small amount with a soft cloth.

To remove light scratches from wood, take a raw walnut (removed from its shell) and rub it on a rough surface to soften the edge then rub the walnut directly on the scratch. It will disappear like magic, and it works on any color of wood.

Lighting

Proper lighting is important for many reasons: performance of visual tasks, regulating the body's circadian system, decreasing fatigue, and improving alertness. It can even affect mood by reducing depression and improving sleep patterns. However, with all of the modern lighting options comes a long list of possible side effects in individuals who have sensitivities to the various components in these lights. Though still a theory, recent studies have suggested that artificial light with a strong blue component could affect human circadian cycles and the hormonal system, and could result in diseases ranging from sleep disorders, immune system disorders, macular degeneration, cardiovascular diseases, diabetes, osteoporosis, and breast cancer.[26] Blue light in particular suppresses melatonin levels almost twice as long as the warmer light alternatives. In some of these conditions, such as epilepsy, migraines, and retinal diseases, it was identified that UV/blue light from artificial sources could make these conditions worse.[27] Natural sunshine provides blue light, but does so at a time when the suppression of melatonin allows for the increased energy and focus you need during the daylight hours. Natural lighting from windows and skylights is the best source for health. Hospitals and office buildings that utilize natural lighting by increasing windows have reported healthier, happier inhabitants as a result.[28] At this point in time, the current consensus on healthy lighting seems to be that natural or blue light during the day and warm light in the afternoons and evenings are ideal. Since electronics like computer monitors, televisions, laptops and smartphone screens all provide blue light, chances are you are receiving more than enough blue light throughout the day. This means it's best for your home lighting in the evening hours to exclude blue light sources when possible.

Because LED lights are very energy efficient they have become a primary source of lighting in most homes, but scientific research is beginning to show some troubling results regarding LED lighting options. Eye health is supported by near-infrared range of light frequency by helping the cells in your retina repair and regenerate, but LED lights have no infrared light, and in fact have an excess of blue light which generates reactive oxygen species (ROS), which may cause damage to DNA and RNA, eventually leading to cell death.[29] In the end, some LED lights are better than others. The easiest on the eyes will have a high Color Rendering Index, or CRI. CRI is the measure in which light sources are graded in their ability to produce natural light. All light has a CRI number: sunlight, for example, has a CRI of 100, as do incandescent light bulbs and candles. The best LED light currently available has a CRI of about 97.[30] Overall, when choosing lights the current choice for the least health risks appears to be warm white incandescent light bulbs.[31] However, the science surrounding bulbs seems to be changing daily, in fact there is a new bulb available called an eco-incandescent bulb. It uses Halogen technology, has a CRI index of 99+, is fully dimmable, mercury free, and meets the federal energy saving requirements. The bulbs are quite affordable at less than $2.00 each and readily available at home improvement stores.

On a side note, wearing blue-blocking Uvex glasses after sun down, especially when viewing computer screens, can be beneficial. There are even apps for your computer and phone screens that can help to reduce the blue light. F.lux is a free app that can be downloaded to your computer, it helps by gradually shifting the screen color to an amber color as the sun sets. During regular daytime hours however your screen will be in the full color spectrum. Once you set it to your time zone, it takes care of the rest. For android phones specifically, there is an app called Twilight. By using your phone's light sensor, Twilight is able to constantly adjust its settings automatically. It progressively reduces the color temperature of the display making it redder, this gradual change means that you barely even notice it happening. The IPhone version 9.3 or newer has a built-in bluelight filter called "night shift"which can be activated in settings.

Wallpaper

You may not think of wallpaper as being unhealthy, but it turns out that it may contribute to an indoor health risk referred to as "sick building syndrome."[32] This syndrome is the result of toxins from fungus growing on the wallpaper becoming airborne. These mycotoxins can be inhaled, causing occupants to feel ill or develop health problems when spending time in certain buildings or homes.[33] The more energy efficient a home is, the more likely it is to aggravate the problem due to the inability to flush out bad air and bring in clean air. Energy efficient houses are better sealed and will just recycle the toxins throughout the home. This is especially true in more humid homes or homes where water using appliances such as coffee makers are used, since damp nooks and crannies create conditions conducive to fungal growth. Another factor is that most traditional wallpapers contain polyvinyl chloride, which leaks Volatile Organic Compounds or VOCs, as well as toxic oil based inks. When these chemicals off-gas, that is, when the chemicals in the material slowly begin to break down and evaporate, they can become airborne and infect your lungs, eyes, nose, and ears.[34]

The Alternatives: There are safe, sustainable wallpapers available, some made from recycled paper, others from renewable sources like bamboo and grasscloth. Most even use natural dyes or nontoxic water based inks. If you are renting and the landlord is unwilling to mitigate the mold problem and moving is not an option there are medical treatments and lifestyle changes that will help one to cope with the health issues caused. Overall, controlling moisture levels in your home is one of the best things you can do to lessen and prevent mold growth.

Unfortunately, even the paste used to apply the wallpaper will off-gas VOCs, and often contains pesticides. There are a few nontoxic wallpaper pastes available online but only from countries outside of the US. When you find a nontoxic wallpaper you like, try making your own paste instead.

Natural wallpaper paste:

- 1 cup **flour**
- 3 tsp **alum**
- **water** as needed
- 10 drops **clove oil**

Combine flour with alum in a double boiler.

Add enough water to make it the consistency of heavy cream.

Heat the mixture while stirring until it thickens to a gravy texture.

Allow it to cool then add the clove oil.

Pour it into a glass container and apply it with a glue brush.

Note: use caution when handling potassium alum; while considered safe by the FDA, it should not be inhaled in powder form and can cause irritation to the skin. Alum is a form of aluminum, and while there are several types, such as potassium alum which is used in pickling and deodorant, all aluminum can be absorbed into your skin.

Smoke Detectors and Fire Alarms

These devices are designed to save lives and they do, but there are some facts that need to be considered before making your purchase. There are two types of smoke detectors, ionizing and photoelectric. According to the NFPA (National Fire Protection Association) ionizing smoke alarms use a radioactive material called americium-241 and are generally more responsive to flaming fires. Photoelectric-based alarms use light instead of alpha and gamma radiation, so when the light is disrupted by the smoke, it sets off the alarm.[35]   The ionizing alarm will respond 30 to 90 seconds faster than the photoelectric alarm if it is detecting fires that originate from petrochemicals like gasoline, which tend to produce flame more quickly, but the alarm can actually take 15 to 50 minutes longer to activate during a smoldering fire and will outright fail to activate up to 20 to 25% of the time in this situation. The photoelectric smoke alarms are quicker to detect the slow-burning, smoldering fires that make up the majority of typical home and office fires. It is recommended that both types be used in the household and there are smoke detectors that combine the two technologies in one unit. What is important when dealing with ionizing smoke detectors however, is proper disposal. If one is crushed or damaged, the small amount of radiation within may leak out and cause health issues. So, when disposing of an old fire alarm, you cannot simply place it in the trash can with your regular waste; you must send it to an official disposal location.

The disposal locations in your area can be found with a quick internet search or by contacting your local fire department. Most often, you will be able to send your old smoke detector through ground mail, but make sure to pack it well and label it fragile so that it does not get crushed or damaged in shipping.

Tile and Popcorn Textured Ceilings

Many homes contain tiles or popcorn texture on the ceiling that contain asbestos and can release toxic fibers. Asbestos was common in ceiling tiles, tile adhesives, dry wall, duct wrap, and ceiling texture sprays up until the 1990s. If breathed in, asbestos fibers can cause mesothelioma or lung cancer.[36] There is no safe level of exposure. Left intact, the materials containing asbestos may not be harmful, however, a thumbtack pushed into a ceiling tile can release thousands of toxic asbestos fibers.[37] If you are not sure whether or not your tiles or ceiling material contains asbestos, there are test kits available or your local state agencies will have up-to-date listings of asbestos experts in your area. If you don't want to expose yourself to the risk, hire an expert. A local asbestos expert can safely remove the tiles or popcorn texture and replace it with a safe water based non-VOC paint.

Paint

Nothing brightens up a room like a fresh coat of paint. However, while the room may look nice, that strong odor left behind contains the toxic VOCs covered earlier. Paint fumes can continue to off-gas in your home for years after painting, so the paint you choose, especially in children's rooms, is very important. There are a few guidelines to help in making the least detrimental paint choices. Select the least toxic, lowest VOC paints available. Look for paints available specifically for children's rooms, with no toxic chemicals, no VOCs, no solvents, and no odor, and it is best to choose water-based over oil-based paint whenever possible. For the absolute lowest VOCs, you can always stick with the base white color, as tints can contain the solvent ethylene glycol and the darker the shade, the higher the level of solvents. Some brands may say "No Odor," yet still contain a high level of VOCs. The label needs to clearly state that it's specially formulated to be low in VOCs. Check the label carefully! Then once you are ready to paint, turn off the air conditioning and cover it with plastic. Keep your windows open and use an exhaust fan. Pregnant people, young children, and pets should stay away from freshly painted rooms for two to three days.

Vacuums

So now that you know about most of the toxins that can be found in your home, in the dust, or brought in from outside, you want to make sure you have a proper device for removing all of that debris from your floor without redistributing it back into the air. To do this you will need a vacuum with a sealed HEPA or S-Class filter. Generally speaking, a bagged vacuum is a better choice for containing the dust collected. They do however tend to lose suction as the bags fill up, and replacing the bags adds to waste and can get expensive. Some models such as Miele and Electrolux have bags that seal themselves as you remove them so that nothing gets into the air. Dyson also makes a vacuum with sealed system HEPA-filtration, but it is bagless, which has its advantages as long as you are not the one emptying it. If, however, you are the person emptying the canister, I would suggest at the very least taking it outside, downwind, and open it over your garbage can. There are sanitizing vacuums like the Verilux CleanWave Sanitizing Portable UV-C Vacuum, which is great for things like upholstery, mattresses, pet beds, and bathroom floors. However, it is hand held and not meant for whole carpets. There is also a vacuum that uses sonic vibrations to loosen the dirt and comes with HEPA sealed filter bags, called the Soniclean VT Plus Upright Vacuum. I hesitate to recommend any one brand, there are many variables to consider: your preferences, specific needs, and budget. But, I do recommend checking the reviews from others who have used the vacuum you are interested in before making the purchase.

Televisions

When I say television can be bad for your health, I am not talking about how far away you need to sit from the screen or even about toxic programing. I'm referring to the unhealthy trend of people sitting for hours on end watching entire seasons of their favorite shows. This type of sedentary lifestyle contributes to a slew of ailments and health issues.[38] One strategy to help prevent this is the TV workout—while watching a television program, commit to getting out of your chair during the commercials. At the very least walk around (it is best to avoid walking to the kitchen for a beer and chips) until your program starts again, but if you are healthy enough for something stronger you can jog in place, do jumping jacks, try the plank position, or jump on a mini trampoline. Even if you are chair bound it is movement that is important because it keeps your circulation going. There are light hand weights or even elastic resistance bands that can be used in a sitting position to strengthen the upper body and ankle weights, or simple leg lifts to strengthen the lower body. Exercise strengthens the immune system, increases energy levels, helps with depression, and can even help you sleep better.[39] Try something different for each commercial break to keep it interesting. By the end of the program you will have most likely spent at least twenty minutes exercising and not taken any time out of your normal routine.

Detoxifying Plants

There are many plants that will remove toxins from the air in your home. NASA did research to see which plants were best for cleaning the air and so would be best for use in space stations; they found that the most efficient air cleaning is accomplished with at least one average sized plant per 100 square feet of home or office space. The following plants were some of their favorites.[40]

Peace Lily: This is a very hardy plant that will grow just about anywhere, even without sunlight. It is a beautiful plant that will produce flowers year-round and can grow quite large depending on the container it is planted in. It is one of the best to remove toxins from your home and absorbs pollutants such as formaldehyde, benzene, and xylene very effectively.[41] Note: if you have animals that enjoy eating houseplants this would not be a good choice, though in general most house plants should be kept away from those animals.

Spider Plant: The spider plant absorbs benzene, formaldehyde, carbon monoxide, and xylene. It too is easy to grow and attractive in your home.

Snake Plant*:* This plant filters benzene, formaldehyde, trichloroethylene, xylene, and toluene.

Aloe Vera*:* While the gel from this plant is fantastic for relieving sunburn (or any burn), it is also a great air purifier. It can serve as a good indicator of how bad the toxins in your home really are because an aloe vera plant will develop brown spots if the level of chemicals it is absorbing has become very high. It does best in a sunny area. Many people like to keep aloe vera plants in their bedrooms because they are said to produce extra oxygen at night which may help people sleep better. The medicinal properties of an aloe vera plant reach maximum potency when the plant is seven years old and stay at that level for the lifetime of the plant.

English Ivy*:* While you may see this plant growing up the sides of buildings or tree trunks, it is unfortunately an invasive species (at least in the Pacific Northwest) that is parasitic to native outdoor plants. However, when planted indoors it filters benzene, formaldehyde, trichloroethylene, xylene, and toluene from the air. It is very hardy, beautiful, and easy to grow.

Bathroom

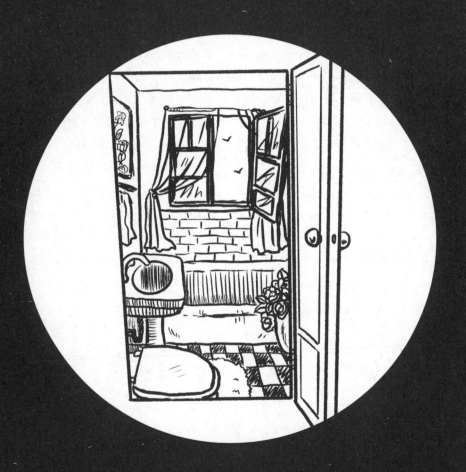

*U*sually the bathroom is the smallest room in the house, but oftentimes it harbors the most toxins. It is important to remember that the largest organ in your body is your skin and that it is very efficient at absorbing the things applied to it. This is the room where most of those things can be found, and they can come from the most unlikely sources. Even your average toilet paper contains dioxins, not that I am asking anyone to give up their soft two ply quilted comfort for plant leaves.[42] When it comes down to it, the healthiest and most environmentally friendly alternative is always a bidet or small shower head that can be easily installed in almost any toilet.

It can be difficult to determine what chemicals or ingredients are in some of these products, even if they are organic, because there are no labeling regulations about natural or organic personal care products, unless you live in California which requires any product labeled organic to have at least 70% organic content. Now, I find this interesting because I had always been under the impression that if something is labeled organic that meant that it was 100% organic . . . Sometimes ignorance is bliss.

Here are some of the toxins you're most likely to run into, and how to replace them.

Cleaners

If you are like most people, you probably have a variety of cleaning products under your bathroom sink. There is a good chance that most, if not all, of these products contain warning labels and the poison control phone number. Add to the fact that they are often used in relatively confined areas and you may need that phone number handy. But remember that most toxic chemicals are accumulative and may take years to show symptoms, and that they are more dangerous to young children and animals. So, you may just want to replace them entirely. Fortunately, this is very easily done with a few basic ingredients. These are all you will need for every cleaning product in your home:

- Baking soda

- White vinegar

- Hydrogen peroxide

- Borax

- Kosher salt

- Castile soap (I like Dr. Bronner's)

- Essential oils (optional)

The best part is that they perform as well or better than the toxic products they are replacing, and all of these products are available in bulk sizes, keeping the cost of your products far below their commercial counterparts.

Toilet cleaner:

- One part **borax**

- Two parts **baking soda**

- 1 cup **vinegar** (adjust as needed)

Mix borax and baking soda together and sprinkle around the toilet.

Spray or pour vinegar over and let it set for about 15 minutes.

Use a brush to scrub and flush the contents.

You can finish by spraying the entire toilet from top to bottom with **hydrogen peroxide** and wiping it down. I also spray the brush used to scrub it with. The toilet will be disinfected, deodorized, and nontoxic. This is an added advantage for those of you who have dogs that insist the only good drinking water is provided by the porcelain drinking bowl.

Window and mirror cleaner:

- ¼ cup **vinegar**

- 3–4 cups **water**

Mix vinegar with water in a spray bottle.

Shake before each use and wipe with a dry cloth.

Another recipe for sparkling windows is to use one tablespoon of **lemon juice** added to one quart of warm **water** in a spray bottle. If the windows are greasy or very dirty you can add a few drops of **castile soap** to either of the above recipes for extra cleaning power. Scratches in glass windows and mirrors can be polished out using **toothpaste** on a soft cloth.

Scouring powder:

Equal parts:

- **Baking soda**

- **Borax**

- **Kosher salt**

Mix equal parts baking soda, borax, and Kosher salt.

Place it all in a shaker bottle and it is ready for use.

You can add several drops of **essential oil** for added fragrance, disinfecting, or cleaning power. Eucalyptus, tea tree, thyme, and lemon oils are all good options for this purpose.

If you would rather purchase a product instead, Bon Ami seems to be the safest alternative at present. However as I have stated before, you must always check the labels for changes in any store-bought products.

Mold and mildew remover: There are two solutions to mold and mildew, the first and my favorite is to simply spray the area affected with **hydrogen peroxide**, wait ten minutes, and wipe the area clean. No rinsing necessary. For more stubborn areas you can make a paste from equal amounts of **borax** and **vinegar**, apply the paste to the area, and allow it to sit for approximately one hour, then rinse the area with **water**.

Drain cleaner: Do I even need to explain how toxic this really is? The main ingredient is usually sulphuric acid mixed with other chemicals that boil up into a toxic cloud, which is easily inhaled and can damage the esophagus and stomach for weeks after exposure. And of course, if you swallow drain cleaner, it can take up to a month for death to occur.[43] Do you really want this in your home? The warning label should include "make sure to complete your bucket list before using." Usually when a bathroom sink or tub becomes clogged, it's due to hair getting trapped in the catch. The easiest solution is a long, spiky, flexible piece of plastic made for this purpose called a drain snake, available at most hardware stores for less than three dollars. While wearing gloves, you simply put the spiky part down the drain and pull out whatever is clogging it. Again, I stress you do this while wearing gloves as it is not only effective but can also be quite disgusting. Another alternative is to pour about a half a cup of **baking soda** down the drain, then add about a cup of **vinegar**. Let it sit for fifteen minutes, then pour a pot of **boiling water** down the drain to finish. Last but not least, there is the plunger—simple and effective. If all else fails, calling a plumber, though expensive, may be less toxic than the chemical alternatives.

Floor cleaner and sanitizer: For both the kitchen and bathroom, just mix about a half a cup of **borax** in a bucket with about two gallons of **hot water** and mop the floor. There is no need to rinse unless you have pets that may lick the floor. This also works well to clean glass shower doors and tracks, but should be rinsed after. While Borax is safer than most cleaning products, it can still be hazardous if inhaled, ingested, or exposed to the skin for a prolonged period of time. Wear gloves if you are not using a mop.

Chrome faucets and grout: An effective and inexpensive way to clean chrome and grout is to apply toothpaste to the surfaces and wipe off. Even an inexpensive store bought brand works for this purpose—it's better on your faucet than in your mouth. For cleaning grout, it is easiest to use an old toothbrush, along with the toothpaste.

Personal Cleaners or Body Care

On average people use about fifteen personal care products every day, and most of these contain chemicals that are carcinogens, neurotoxins, and may contain hormone disruptors.[44] A friend of mine jokingly compared all the chemicals we are exposed to on a daily basis to death by a thousand cuts. Even in trace amounts these toxins can accumulate in our bodies. Combined with other sources we are exposed to it can become a chemical nightmare. Toothpaste, deodorant, and even your soap are just a few examples of the unsuspected sources containing toxins you may encounter on a daily basis.

Face cleaner and makeup remover: To avoid the alcohols, preservatives, and formaldehyde-releasing chemicals in these products, a simple solution is to use **coconut oil** instead. It is antibacterial, antifungal, and an excellent moisturizer without clogging your pores. It is safe and effective for use around your eyes, and can even help minimize those fine lines that can form from all the extra smiling you'll be doing.[45] Coconut oil is known for its anti-aging properties due mostly to the three fatty acids, saturated, monounsaturated and polyunsaturated fats, naturally occurring vitamin-E, and proteins which help to repair and rejuvenate the skin. In some cases coconut oil can even be good for acne prone skin, battling the microbial bodies and healing the affected skin.[46] To clean your skin or remove your makeup with **coconut oil,** just take a small amount of oil and rub it between your palms, then gently apply it to your face and in a circular motion around your eyes. Then take a warm wet washcloth and lay it on your face. Leave it for a moment, then gently wipe away the oil. Follow with toner (below) and moisturizer of your choice. At night, simply use a small amount of coconut oil then take a drop of castor oil rubbed between your fingers and add it to your eyelashes, eyebrows, and lips.

Toner: Most toners are alcohol based and can be very drying to your skin. They can also throw off the natural pH balance of your skin and can contain the usual chemical culprits such as phthalates, parabens, and formaldehyde-releasing DMDM hydantoin. A much easier and safer solution is to pour a small amount of **aloe vera gel** onto a cotton pad and go over your face, allow it to dry, and moisturize. Note that many products advertising as aloe vera gels do not in fact contain any aloe vera. As always, check the ingredients list. My personal choice is Lily of the Desert Organic Aloe Vera Gel. Another option would be to make a mixture of one part organic **apple cider vinegar** with two parts distilled or purified **water**.

Shake before adding it to a cotton pad and go over your face, no need to rinse, simply moisturize as usual. Apple cider vinegar is especially good for restoring the natural pH of acne prone or oily skin.[47]

Face and body scrubs: Body scrubs are used to exfoliate dead skin and stimulate collagen production to improve the condition and appearance of your skin. These scrubs usually contain microbeads, which are tiny plastic pellets so small they get rinsed right down the bathroom drain and travel right through wastewater treatment plants. These plastic beads are made from oil, and are not biodegradable, so when they end up in the water they absorb any toxic pollution and become even more dangerous. They then make their way up the food chain, and back to us. A report by the Joint Group of Experts on the Scientific Aspects of Marine Environmental Protection states that people who eat a lot of shellfish seafood could be unwittingly consuming thousands of microbeads every year, with 25% of commercially processed fish in the US containing microplastics.[48] In addition to microbeads, these body scrubs can also contain other toxic culprits like synthetic fragrances, parabens, phthalates, and other words that no one can pronounce without a degree in chemistry. A simple solution to replace these scrubs would be to mix equal amounts of **coconut oil** and **baking soda**—it's quick, simple, and very effective. It works as an exfoliant and helps to reduce age spots and restore a healthy glow to your face, and can be used all over your body and rinsed off in the shower to leave you with smooth moisturized skin.[49] If you want to make a cellulite reducing scrub simply replace the baking soda with **coffee grounds**, which will help reduce the appearance of cellulite and the antioxidants in the coffee will increase collagen production.[50] The effects can last about a week. Another very effective way to exfoliate your skin is dry skin brushing. It has also been claimed that dry brushing may stimulate the lymphatic system, increase blood flow, and further rid your body of toxins.[51] All you need for this is a natural bristle brush and a few extra minutes before you shower. It is very simple to do: you start with your feet and *lightly* brush your skin in short sweeping motions toward your heart. Continue up both legs then go on to your arms, starting with your fingers, always towards your heart. Then you can finish with your stomach and back in circular motions towards your heart. Keep the strokes light. It should never hurt but instead leave your skin tingly and refreshed. Finish with a nice shower and moisturize with a little coconut oil from head to toe.

Remember when exfoliating to do so gently, and limit it to three times a week or less. Calluses are formed as the body's natural defense to the constant rubbing of an area. Excessive exfoliation can lead to rough and thickened skin.

Anti-acne face mask: You can avoid the expense and toxic chemicals of all the drug store products promising smoother, clearer skin by mixing a few simple ingredients at home:

- 1 tbsp **coconut oil**

- 1 tbsp **baking soda**

- ½ capsule **activated charcoal**

Mix together ingredients until thoroughly mixed.

Apply the paste to your face.

Let it sit for about five minutes, then rinse completely.

Pat your face dry with a towel.

Finish by toning with **apple cider vinegar** on a cotton pad. This will help to correct the pH balance of your skin. Note that activated charcoal may stain clothing.

Soaps and shampoos*:* These products contain too many toxins to list, but a few you might be familiar with are sodium lauryl sulfate, triclosan, formaldehyde, and toluene. Most shampoos, styling products, cream rinses, and shaving products contain parabens. They go by many names such as methylparaben, ethylparaben, or propylparaben, and while these were once thought to be safe they are now being linked to various cancers due to their hormone disrupting properties.[52] They are absorbed even more aggressively when alcohol is also present in the ingredient list. Here's the amazing part: these toxic chemicals can even be found in baby shampoos. Anything with added fragrance will most likely contain phthalates which have been shown to disrupt hormones. Retinyl palmitate, a synthetic form of palm oil, is listed as a probable carcinogen and is also found in most shampoos and personal care products. On their website, The Campaign for Safe Cosmetics lists DEA (Diethanolamine), MEA (Monoethanolamine), and TEA (triethanolamine) as three more hormone disrupting chemicals to watch out for, due to the fact that they can form cancer causing agents.[53] These can be found in just about any cosmetic or personal care product.

The list goes on and it can be difficult to keep up with the latest research on what may kill you this week. My general rule of thumb is not to put anything *on* my body that I wouldn't put *in* my body. That being said, I do use Dr. Bronners bar soap but do not think I would enjoy eating it. Fortunately there are many safe shampoos on the market, though admittedly they are usually sold in health food stores or online. There is always diluted **liquid castile soap**, but depending on your hair type it can leave it dry and frizzy. One way to prevent that is to mix equal parts liquid **castile soap** and **coconut milk** in a bottle, shake it before each use, and shampoo as usual. Another alternative is to mix one teaspoon **baking soda** with one cup of **water** in a squeeze bottle and work it into your hair, starting from the roots through to the ends. Let it sit for a few minutes, then rinse with cool water. Last, use this vinegar rinse to finish:

- One part **apple cider vinegar**

- Four parts **water**

Mix one part **apple cider vinegar** to four parts water in a squeeze bottle.

Rinse through your hair, avoiding your eyes.

This makes an effective clarifying shampoo, and your hair will be shiny and feel thicker. The great part about making your own shampoo is that you can tailor it to the needs of your hair at that particular time. For example, if you start with the basic **one teaspoon baking soda** to one **cup of water,** you can add a few drops of **olive oil, coconut oil,** or **jojoba oil** if your hair is too dry. If it is feeling too oily or if there is build up from other products, you can add a few drops of **castile soap** to the baking soda base. Baking soda exfoliates your hair and removes the extra sebum, using it together with an apple cider vinegar rinse restores the natural pH balance of the hair shaft. It should be noted that the first time you use baking soda and vinegar your hair may appear dull and waxy, however after a few more washes you should start to notice healthy shiny hair. Some people even experience thicker growth as a result of the removal of excess sebum which can restrict growth and increase hair loss.[54]

Hair gels and creams: I have long naturally curly hair with a mind of its own and I have found after many years of trying to control it that it is best to let it have its own way about where it wants to part or how much it wants to curl. I have also learned, through trial and error, how to prevent it from becoming a giant frizzy mass. In place of hair gel, I use **aloe vera**: just pour the appropriate amount for your length of hair into your hands and scrunch it into the curls. Then I use a diffuser attachment on my blowdryer to dry my hair, but just before it is fully dried I add a home made **oil mixture**:

- Jojoba oil

- Castor oil

- Melted coconut oil

- Argan oil

- A little bit of Vitamin E

Combine equal amounts of jojoba oil, castor oil, melted coconut oil, argan oil, and a little vitamin E oil in a squeeze bottle. Vitamin E oil makes a great natural preservative so your products will last longer.

Add two drops of essential oil for fragrance.

Shake before use and pour about a dime size or less depending on length in your hand.

Rub your hands together, scrunch into the nearly dried curls, and you have healthy fragrant hair. As for how much of each of the oils goes into making the mixture, I have to admit to just squirting some of each from the original bottles. I never measure, but it doesn't seem to make a lot of difference. I always try to buy organic sources when purchasing the oils and I stock up when I find them on sale. It should be said however, that even at their regular price, the cost of making it yourself is far cheaper than the store-bought version. If you have straight or fine hair you can use the same products but use much less. If you need a product to help thicken your hair you can use two parts **castor oil** mixed with one part melted **coconut oil**, and massage that into your scalp when you go to bed at night. You do not need to thoroughly coat the hair, it's really the scalp you are applying it to, although your hair will also benefit. If you use a small amount you will not need to protect your pillow. If, however, you are using it as a conditioning treatment and coating your hair you will want to cover your pillow and you will need to wash your hair the next morning. On a side note, **castor oil**, when applied to eyelashes and eyebrows, helps to thicken them both. So, at the end of the day when you wash your face, I recommend using **coconut oil** to remove makeup and dirt, then you can apply a little castor oil to your eyelashes and eyebrows. The coconut oil moisturizes your skin and the castor oil helps hydrate and nourish lashes to prevent breakage and stimulate new growth.[55] It doesn't take much castor oil to do the trick, and if you get it in your eyes, don't worry. It is actually good for your eyes and is used as a safe alternative for eye drops in people who suffer from dry eyes. Any castor oil left on your hands can be rubbed into your cuticles or onto your lips to prevent cracking. Again, as a reminder I always recommend using organic sources for the products you are using.

Hair coloring and dyes: I always thought nature provided us with the best hair color for our skin tone. At least that is what I believed until I hit 30, and then nature and I disagreed on when I should start to get gray hair. I was determined to dye my hair as close to my natural color as possible, however my research into hair dyes was very troubling. It turns out hair color may be a contributing factor to certain serious health risks.[56] Common ingredients such as PPD (para-phenylenediamine) and a similar compound,

PTD, were linked to cancer, rheumatoid arthritis, and allergic reactions. In fact, a study done at the University of Southern California found that women who colored their hair once a month for fifteen years or more had twice the risk of contracting bladder cancer than non-users.[57] Even the so called "natural" or "organic" hair dyes contain ingredients that can be harmful. Check the ingredient list on the package. While any natural or organic ingredients will be in big bold letters you may still find the toxic ones listed in small print on the back. The exception to this is Henna. Henna is a nontoxic alternative to color your hair and will even cover gray. It does have its drawbacks: it can not lighten your hair, is not as easy to apply as regular hair coloring, and will add a bit of red tones to your normal color. It will temporarily cover gray but tends to fade after several washes leaving the once gray areas a dark orange hue. On the positive side, besides being safe to use, it will add shine and make your hair feel fuller. I have tried some homemade versions of hair dyes such as coffee, black tea and black walnut powder, with little success. This may be because I am trying to cover the gray and that is a bit more difficult than just coloring your hair. On a final note, if you must use hair dyes, try to choose the least toxic versions, keep it off of your scalp as much as possible, drink lots of water before, during, and after the coloring process, and make sure you rinse it out completely (preferably not in the shower, where it coats your body on the way down the drain). Some people are so sensitive to the toxic chemicals in hair dyes that they become sick after each application and find it necessary to use a sauna or soak in a detox bath of Epsom salts and baking soda for relief.[58] I try to limit how often I dye my hair and when I do, I only apply a quarter of the bottle at a time to cover the new growth. I use a fan artist brush, dip the end in the dye, and place it at the base of the hairline, avoiding the scalp as much as possible. If you are pregnant, it's better to just avoid hair dye altogether. Your baby will thank you for it.

Makeup and Cosmetics

Like hair dyes, makeup products from lipstick to mascara are full of ingredients that would be dangerous to handle in large quantities. Did you know that one out of every eight of the 82,000 possible ingredients used to create beauty products are actually industrial chemicals? They include known carcinogens, pesticides, reproductive toxins, hormone disruptors, degreasers, and plasticizers.[59] The good news is that there are beauty products available, usually in health food stores or online, that are striving to provide safer alternatives. There is even a verification process available to consumers who want to know about the safety of the ingredients in these more natural alternatives, and there is currently a website (ewg.org/ewgverified) where you can check over 900 products and their safety ratings. The Environmental Working Group (EWG) is a nonprofit, non-partisan, independent organization dedicated to protecting human life and the environment. They have a team of scientists that do groundbreaking research and then provide reports and online databases to educate consumers on making safer and more informed choices about the products they buy and the companies they support. When you take good care of your health, chances are your skin will be clear, your eyes bright, and your hair shiny, but if nature needs a little help try the less toxic products, or even make your own.

Eyeliner: A very effective eyeliner can be made from emptying a capsule of **activated charcoal** into a small glass container and adding a drop or two of distilled water, mix well, and apply with a fine brush. If left in the powder form the activated charcoal provides a smoky effect as an eyeshadow. It takes some experimenting to get the desired effect so I do not recommend using it for the first time if you are in a hurry to get somewhere. It is not waterproof which goes without saying. If you get any in your eyes, rinse it thoroughly and see a doctor if irritation continues. And remember that activated charcoal can stain clothing.

Lip gloss: Castor oil or coconut oil are great alternatives to conventional lip gloss or, for less shine, you can use food grade organic cocoa butter or shea butter. If you prefer tinted lip gloss you can add herbal powders such as powdered hibiscus or natural red food coloring to any of the oils or butters or even a combination thereof. It all depends on your preferences.

Foundation: Instead of store bought foundation, try using rosehip seed oil or moringa oil to keep your skin smooth and blemish free. Rosehip oil protects the skin, is very healing and has regenerative properties that provide anti-aging benefits. It also stimulates collagen production and helps protect against sun damage.[60]

Cold-pressed rosehip seed oil is the best option because it retains more nutrients than the heated version, but it is more expensive. Moringa oil helps to eliminate inflammation, slows the aging process by reducing oxidative stress, and is exceedingly moisturizing.[61]

Nail polish: You may be surprised to hear that the toxic chemicals in your nail polish show up in your body. Researchers found that about ten hours after nail polish was applied to the participants in their study, everyone showed increased levels of DPHP, a chemical produced when the body metabolizes Triphenyl phosphate (TPHP), the chemical in the nail polish, once again proving that what goes *on* your body goes *in* your body. TPHP toxicity studies in animals shows that it can alter sex hormone balance, reproductive performance, and impact metabolic function and weight gain.[62, 63] The very few human studies done have shown that it alters endocrine function, impacts reproduction, alters thyroid levels and decreases semen quality.[64] This is further backed up by numerous animal studies.[65] So, if you choose to use nail polish it is best to opt for the least toxic, TPHP, and formaldehyde free versions. They are available almost everywhere, but you have to read the labels. If you just want your nails to look nice and be healthy, the options include an inexpensive buffing block or chamois buffer. Both will leave your nails shiny, and the buffing action stimulates healthy nail growth. Keep the cuticles moisturized with coconut, jojoba, or castor oil.

Deodorant and Antiperspirant: Deodorant was first introduced in 1888, and many people felt that it was unnecessary, especially those who lived in rural areas and worked outdoors. However, by the early 1900's cities were thriving and more and more people started moving to populated areas and working in factories, stores, and offices. Working so closely together, people soon realized the need for deodorant not only for themselves but for their coworkers. If you couldn't afford the .25 cent price tag to purchase a jar of deodorant you could make your own with a recipe from an article in the Los Angeles Times health and beauty section (Sept. 13th, 1903).[66] Unfortunately, it called for carbolic acid, alcohol, corn starch, powdered orris, essence of iris, and glycerin. The carbolic acid would cause chemical burns, and when mixed together with the other ingredients looked like peanut butter, but reportedly smelled pleasant. Deodorant works by killing bacteria, however it is important to remember that there are good bacteria and bad bacteria. By killing the bacteria you also lose the beneficial microbes that help to balance the pH of the underarm environment and prevent offensive odors.[67] Antiperspirant followed in 1903, developed by a surgeon to keep his hands from sweating during surgery.[68] Antiperspirant contains aluminum, which works by reacting with sweat to form a plug over the sweat glands and thereby preventing any sweat from escaping.[69] Thanks to advertising aimed at targeting insecurities, deodorant and antiperspirant sales reached one million dollars by 1927, and the industry is worth over 18 billion today. Keep in mind that the body is an amazingly efficient machine when allowed to work the way it was intended. There is a reason we perspire, it helps the body regulate temperature as well as helping it to eliminate toxins. Studies have shown that sweat contains heavy metals such as arsenic, cadmium, lead, and mercury that are all being removed from the body.[70] You do not want these heavy metals to stay in your body. This is the reason people use saunas, and indigenous people the world over have regularly visited sweat lodges for detoxification. To add insult to injury, antiperspirants usually contain aluminum salts, which research suggests has a genotoxic profile that accumulates in breast tissue, causing cancer by altering DNA and interfering with estrogen receptors.[71, 72] Most people use these products daily, and in a sensitive area known to absorb the products applied, so you need to be mindful of what you are applying. An easy nontoxic solution is to use a little organic coconut oil under each arm, and if necessary finish by sprinkling a little baking soda for good measure. Coconut oil is naturally antibacterial, antifungal, and smells great. If you decide you need something a little stronger you can make your own safe, personalized deodorant using:

- ¼ cup of **baking soda**

- ¼ cup of organic **coconut oil**

- ¾ cup **cornstarch**

- A few drops of your favorite essential oils—like thyme—to really boost effectiveness

Mix together in a small glass jar with a nice label and you are all set.

Perfume and Aftershave: Synthetic fragrances contain a high number of toxic chemicals, most of which are not even listed on the label. They are protected as "trade secrets." These fragrances can be found in almost all personal products like shampoo, soap, lotion, deodorant, and, of course, perfume and aftershave. Organic **essential oils** or 100% naturally derived fragrances are a safer option for a pleasing scent. You can create your own individual scent by mixing a few of your favorite oils together and then diluting them in a carrier oil. The carrier oil you choose depends on the product you are adding the scent to. For example, avocado oil or almond oil is very moisturizing; coconut oil, olive oil, and jojoba is great in just about anything but particularly beneficial in hair products. Just remember what you chose so that you can replicate it again when needed. You can then add this personal scent to your homemade products without having to worry about conflicting scents from multiple products. Be mindful that they can still cause allergic reactions and other issues for people who are particularly sensitive to fragrances.

Shaving cream: Used on large areas of the body, shaving cream is easily absorbed into your skin and is another source of toxic chemicals we've talked about, like TEA, DEA, and MEA to name just a few of the many culprits. They are hormone disruptors and form carcinogenic nitrates and nitrosamines.[73] The good news is that there are some great safe alternatives, my favorite being Dr. Bronner's Shaving Gel. Or, you can make your own:

- Mix equal amounts of **shea butter** and **coconut oil**

- Add a few drops of **vitamin E oil**, and, if desired, essential oils.

- Store in a labeled glass container so that you do not confuse it with your homemade deodorant.

This is a very moisturizing and healing mixture. If you want a foaming shaving cream, you can mix one quarter cup each of **castile soap**, **aloe vera** gel, and **water** in a bottle, add one tablespoon **almond oil** and **vitamin E**, and shake before each use.

Toothpaste: The inside lining of your mouth can absorb a large percentage of what it comes in contact with, and this includes any potentially hazardous chemicals or carcinogens and impurities.[74] Even if you read the label to protect yourself from known toxins, manufacturers don't have to list all the ingredients on their packaging. You may find some of the following in your favorite brand of toothpaste:

- *Carrageenan*: An unnecessary ingredient that causes gastrointestinal inflammation, and higher rates of colon cancer, in laboratory animals.[75]

- *Triclosan*: In animal studies, levels of thyroid hormone and testosterone were affected as well as endocrine disrupting activity. These studies also found decreased cardiovascular functions, reproductive and developmental defects, and allergies and asthma, while animal studies show it can interfere with brain and reproductive system functioning.[76]

- *Propylene glycol*: While toxic levels of exposure are rare, it is a known skin irritant and is the active ingredient in engine coolants and antifreeze.[77]

You may even see some of these ingredients in "natural" toothpaste. This is only a partial list and doesn't even include the many dyes used, a source of heavy metals like aluminum, chromium, and barium.

The Alternatives: So, what can you do instead? Well, once again Dr. Bronner's makes a very nice nontoxic toothpaste available in stores, but there are also other options available for healthy oral care. **Oil pulling** is a technique used for centuries in many parts of the world to prevent tooth decay, heal and strengthen gums, whiten teeth, and eliminate bad breath.[78] Oil pulling is safe, and an effective way to draw toxins out of your mouth, and some say even your body. Oil pulling can be done with any oil, but in order to prevent absorbing any unwanted chemicals from processing make sure to choose a high quality **organic oil** such as coconut oil in a glass jar. It is best when done first thing in the morning before you brush your teeth, and is very easy to do. You simply take about two to three teaspoons of your preferred oil, let's say coconut, and swish it around your mouth for about 10 to 20 minutes. After swishing the oil around for about 20 minutes you will want to spit it into the trash as it could potentially clog the sink. At this point you can finish by gently brushing your teeth. On a final note, oil pulling is not recommended for young children due to the potential choking hazard in the event they accidentally swallow it. You can make your own toothpaste by combining one quarter cup of **coconut oil** with one quarter cup of food grade **diatomaceous earth** or **baking soda**, then add a few drops of **organic peppermint flavoring** and powdered **xylitol** to taste. Take care not to inhale the **diatomaceous earth** which can cause respiratory irritation. Customize your toothpaste to serve your needs by starting with that base and adding any of the following items depending on your preference and conditions:

- **Activated charcoal**: a whitening agent

- **Peppermint** flavoring, **cinnamon**, or **orange** flavoring: to add desired flavors. Simply Organic has a line of flavoring to choose from

- **Xylitol powder**: a sweetener, antibacterial, helps pH balance[79]

- **Baking soda**: mildly abrasive, some whitening effect[80]

- **Diatomaceous earth**: mildly abrasive, contains healthy trace minerals

- **Coconut oil**: helps reduce cavity causing bacteria, prevents candida in the mouth[81]

- **Trace mineral drops**: helps to remineralize tooth enamel (Note: very little needed)[82]

- **Bentonite clay**: natural tooth polisher, rich in minerals, reduces mouth acidity.[83]

As an example, if I were making a toothpaste for a child I would use the coconut oil, baking soda mixture, and add a couple drops of trace minerals, orange flavoring, and xylitol powder. It would taste good, clean the teeth well, and be nontoxic if swallowed.

Remember that when brushing your teeth, it is recommended that you spend about two minutes, using a soft-bristled brush, gently cleaning all the surfaces of your teeth. Excessive pressure while brushing can cause issues with your gums.

Raw Organic Cacao Nibs: These are a great substitute for those times when you can't brush as cacao has been shown to reduce tooth decay by suppressing the bacteria that causes plaque.[84] Besides tasting good they are low in calories, high in fiber, loaded with antioxidants, contain phytonutrients, and are said to enhance one's mood and energy.

Mouthwash: Your body is amazing. When allowed to work the way intended it keeps you healthy and protects you from disease. Your mouth, for example contains special good bacteria that promotes proper digestion and blood vessel health. Most mouthwashes contain the chemical chlorhexidine, which destroys these good bacteria and weakens the immune system. If you are looking for a safe mouthwash to purchase, look for alcohol-free brands made from **glycerin**, **aloe vera**, and **essential oils**. Better yet, a two part water to one part mixture of 3% concentration of **hydrogen peroxide** with a few drops of **peppermint flavoring** will not only freshen your breath but help to whiten your teeth. Make sure not to swallow though, as ingesting hydrogen peroxide can, if undiluted, burn internal organs and cause internal bleeding. Even when diluted, ingesting hydrogen peroxide can still result in mild stomach pain.

Dental floss: Yes, even your basic dental floss can contain a chemical that has been classified as a potential carcinogen, thanks to the chemical used in place of natural wax. The perfluorinated polymer (PFC) used interferes with hormone and immune function, while teflon, another chemical used to coat floss, has also been found to be highly toxic.[85] There are safe alternatives in floss available that do not use this toxin but it is important to read the ingredient label. As mentioned before, even then you are not always assured that it does *not* contain certain ingredients, as the manufacturers are not required to disclose all of the ingredients. The safe brands will usually state that they are free of petro-wax and synthetic chemicals. My personal favorite is a brand that uses organic silk. Another alternative would be a water flosser though caution should be used in how strong the water stream is set as this can cause damage to the gums if it is too high.

Teeth whiteners: I am admittedly addicted to chocolate and coffee. Though I do limit myself to one cup of coffee a day, it is not exactly your standard eight-ounce cup, it's more of a large mug requiring two hands. After all, coffee can be good for you in moderation: it is full of antioxidants, protects against cirrhosis of the liver, and lowers your risk for type two diabetes.[86] As for chocolate, I make a daily cup of hot cocoa from organic raw cacao, and while it is a healthy superfood full of nutrition, it can also be a nightmare for staining teeth. Between the coffee and cacao, my teeth were less than pearly white. But I am not willing to use the standard protocol for whitening teeth. Just reading the warning labels should be enough to make you think twice before using one of these products, not to mention the tooth sensitivity and irritated gums sometimes resulting from the procedure. Luckily, there are quite a few natural alternatives to pick from. Oil pulling alone has a whitening effect on teeth when done on a daily basis, however, when used in combination with activated charcoal and baking soda the effect is impressive. To do this just oil pull as usual, then when you are finished and ready to brush your teeth dip your rinsed toothbrush into a mixture of equal parts **activated charcoal** and **baking soda** (I keep a small amount premixed in a glass container). At this point you can add a small amount of nontoxic toothpaste to the toothbrush to help with the consistency, and gently brush, do not scrub your teeth. The baking soda is mildly abrasive and the activated charcoal removes stains and bacteria. While you are brushing your teeth, they will look black and scary but I assure you this is temporary. Once you have finished brushing you can rinse with a mouthwash made from **hydrogen peroxide** slightly diluted with **warm water**. I use a small shot glass about three quarters full of hydrogen peroxide and about one quarter water and rinse about thirty seconds. Then fill the shot glass with plain water and rinse again to remove the hydrogen peroxide. Your pearly whites will look and feel like you just had them cleaned at the dentist office except without the sensitivity. You can do this on a daily basis to keep your teeth at their whitest, just remember to brush gently to avoid irritating your gums. If you accidentally ingest any of these ingredients please note the following:

Activated charcoal, while taken internally by many to aid with digestion and used in Emergency rooms to treat accidental poisoning, can interfere with many medications including birth control due to its ability to absorb the chemicals involved and pass them through the intestines. Baking soda is used internally by many to de-acidify their bodies and is safe if swallowed. Hydrogen peroxide should not be swallowed as it can upset your stomach.

Medicine Cabinet

Talcum powder: There is a lot of controversy surrounding talcum powder and cancer risks. For now, the International Agency for Research on Cancer considers talc-containing products as "possibly carcinogenic to humans,"[87] and The American Academy of Pediatrics advises against using talcum baby powder on babies due to possible aspiration risks.[88] That's enough for me to choose organic or non-GMO **corn starch** as a great natural alternative. **Baking soda** also works just as well and is very cost effective. Both work very well for any applications for which you would typically use talcum powder, although I am told that baking soda works best for sprinkling inside of sneakers to prevent odors and moisture.

Sunscreen: The sun is essential for life: it provides natural vitamin D and helps to regulate your melatonin levels for a proper wake/sleep cycle. There are three types of rays produced by the sun: UVA, UVC, and UVB. The ozone filters out all of the UVC and allows only 10% of the UVB and 95% of the UVA to reach the earth's surface.[89] Only the UVB rays will produce vitamin D, and while they only penetrate the outer layer of skin, they are the ones responsible for sunburn and are linked to skin cancer. UVA penetrates deeper into the skin, is instrumental in skin damage causing premature aging and wrinkles, and is present during all daylight hours due to its ability to penetrate clouds and windows. UVA damages

DNA which can eventually lead to cancer.[90] Spray-on sunscreens can be particularly bad for children because they can release toxic nanoparticles into the air that can be harmful when inhaled. Added to that, spray-on sunscreens are a poor choice because they are less likely to be properly applied to the skin, defeating the whole point of your beach ritual. The list goes on. The worst part? Many sunscreens only protect against UVB rays, allowing the dangerous UVA rays through.

The Alternatives:

- 1/3 cup **coconut oil**, which has a natural SPF of approximately 10 to 20

- 10 to 30 drops of **Myrrh oil**, SPF of approximately 15

- ½ cup of **Shea butter**, SPF of approximately 5 to 6

Some people like to add two tablespoons of **zinc oxide**, which has an SPF of 30+. If you do choose to add zinc oxide, make sure to use **non-nano zinc**. The reason for this is that while the nanoparticles are more transparent they offer less UVA protection. Nanoparticles can also be inhaled into the lungs and thereby enter the bloodstream. Zinc oxide provides a broad spectrum of protection for both UVB and UVA rays. I recommend wearing a mask when mixing it to avoid inhaling any.[91]

Aloe vera juice or gel also provides some SPF protection and is particularly good for healing sunburned skin.[92]

The other safe alternatives are preventatives: a good hat, long sleeved shirts, and common sense.

Hand sanitizer: A staple for on-the-go parents, hand sanitizer is seen as a godsend at public play areas or fast food restaurants to help protect children from the latest colds, flu, or currently shared viruses. Most classrooms require them in an effort to thwart student absenteeism from illnesses. Unfortunately, it turns out hand sanitizers can potentially cause some bacteria to become alcohol tolerant, and often contains chemicals such as triclosan or triclocarban that can lead to damage to the outer protective layer of skin cells, reproductive issues, and is an endocrine disruptor.[93] Triclosan kills off the good bacteria but allows the bad, antibiotic-resistant bacteria to grow. If that's not enough, studies have confirmed that hand sanitizers in general increase your skin's ability to absorb the dangerous chemical bisphenol A (BPA),[94] a chemical linked to hormone disorders, cancer, heart disease, and diabetes. Most BPA exposure comes from food and beverage packaging, however many people may not realize that receipt paper is coated with high levels of the chemical. To make matters worse, after using hand sanitizer your skin's ability to absorb BPA increases by 100-fold.[95] So using hand sanitizer at a fast food restaurant and then taking the receipt in hand for the purchase transfers the BPA to the food to be eaten as well as being absorbed by your skin. The fact is that hand sanitizers are a convenient alternative when you cannot wash your hands with soap and water, especially during flu season, but there are a number of safe alternatives available in your local health food store. Make sure to always read the labels before you choose one. Look for plant based ingredients and essential oils. You can make an alcohol free nontoxic version that will do the job as well:

- A couple ounces of (alcohol free) **witch hazel**

- 4 ounces **aloe vera**

- 5 drops **tea tree oil**

- A few drops of **eucalyptus** and **vitamin E oil**

- Mix witch hazel with about aloe vera.

- Add tea tree oil, eucalyptus oil, and Vitamin E oil.

- Place it all in a small squeeze bottle and you are all set.

Another very easy alternative is to simply keep a small spray bottle of **hydrogen peroxide,** spray it on your hands, and shake them dry.

Triple Antibiotic Ointment: A favorite among many for cuts and scrapes, antibiotic ointments like Neosporin have been around since the 1950's. Some people swear by its healing abilities and say they have used it all their life with no ill effects. Unfortunately, a recent study shows that triple antibiotic ointment may be contributing to the spread of MRSA.[96] However, there are natural alternatives you can use instead. How about something that has been around for thousands of years and is considered by some to be more effective than antibacterial creams with no side effects? Honey, especially raw manuka honey, has incredible benefits. It has been used to successfully treat MRSA bacteria, and when used as a wound dressing it promotes rapid healing and prevents infection.[97] Honey reduces pain and inflammation and stimulates the production of cells that aid in the repair of tissue damage. It is also very effective for use on burns. Of course, if you are allergic to bees you should use caution when using any honey products. Note: Honey should never be given to babies under one year of age for risk of botulism. If honey is not an option for you for any reason, you can make your own alternative. This is my favorite version of triple antibiotic ointment, I always keep a small container in my backpack for cuts and scrapes:

- 3 tbsp **coconut oil**

- 1 tbsp **pure beeswax**

• 5 drops **oregano**, **thyme**, and **tea tree essential oils**

Mix coconut oil and pure beeswax in a double boiler until it liquifies together.

Remove it from the heat and add oregano, thyme, and tea tree essential oils.

Stir and pour into a small labeled glass container.

Hemorrhoid cream: Most commercial hemorrhoid creams use petroleum or petroleum jelly as a base, then add mineral oil and parabens. Preventing hemorrhoids in the first place is a great first step, and some things that will aid in that goal is to eat a healthy, fiber rich diet, drink plenty of water, exercise regularly, and consider using a step stool placed in front of your toilet to help correct your posture when answering the call of nature. When your knees are elevated it creates a squatting position and reduces the strain that can cause hemorrhoids by aligning everything for easier and more complete elimination. As for diet, many have had success by adding probiotics and fermented foods such as sauerkraut, yogurt, and miso to their menus. There are many causes of hemorrhoids and some are unavoidable. Stress, pregnancy, prolonged sitting, diet, and even biblical plagues have all been blamed for this painful and irritating malady. A nice twenty minute "sitz bath," followed by aloe vera gel or witch hazel applied to the affected area usually brings relief. Fill a small plastic tub that fits over a toilet seat with warm water and Epsom salt, using a solution of 1/4 cup of epsom salt per 4 cups of warm water. Mix the water until all of the salt is dissolved and sit in the shallow bath. Another home remedy is to mix two tablespoons of epsom salts with two tablespoons of glycerin. Apply this mixture to a gauze pad, then place the pad on the painful area and leave it in place for about twenty minutes. Some people swear by using a (peeled) garlic clove suppository once or twice a day to heal the affected area. Or for an extra strength version you can try a combination of garlic, witch hazel, and coconut oil. Garlic reinforces blood vessels, reduces inflammation, and has antibiotic effects, and when combined with witch hazel and coconut oil it makes an effective suppository. Some research indicates that witch hazel may shrink swollen veins and reduce itching while coconut oil promotes healing, is anti-inflammatory, and provides a base and lubrication for the suppository.[98]

Hemorrhoid suppository:

- 3 cloves **garlic**
- ¼ cup organic **coconut oil**
- 10 drops of (alcohol free) **witch hazel**
- A few drops **aloe vera** gel
- Using a garlic press crush 3 cloves of fresh organic **garlic** into a bowl.

Add ¼ cup of organic **coconut oil**, 10 drops of (alcohol free) **witch hazel**, and a few drops of **aloe vera** gel.

Mix well and place small amounts in a suppository shape onto a piece of parchment or wax paper.

Refrigerate for at least 20 minutes before use and keep stored in the refrigerator.

Insert one suppository into your anus at bedtime so that it can work overnight.

Note: you may feel a burning sensation at first from the garlic but this should subside. If it continues to be a problem you can use less garlic in your preparation.

If you prefer, a single clove of garlic can be peeled and used as a suppository by itself.

These homemade suggestions are only alternatives to over-the-counter products used for these conditions. If your hemorrhoids are bleeding and causing severe pain, you should seek medical advice.

Bug repellant: We have all heard about how toxic DEET is, but it is even worse when combined with the other chemicals used in insecticides. This mixture then becomes toxic to the central nervous system. It has been found to cause issues with motor skills, memory and behavior problems, tremors, and for some, can even cause seizures.[99, 100] On the other hand, the true essential oil of lemon eucalyptus is often used instead, which can be very effective, but may be dangerous for use on children under three years of age since it can cause skin and eye irritation.. There's also catnip oil, which has been shown to be more effective than DEET.[101] It is important to avoid ticks and mosquitoes and the diseases they carry during the summer months, especially for your children, so here are a few options for a safe effective bug repellent spray:

- ½ cup **apple cider vinegar**

- ½ cup **witch hazel**

- 10 drops: **citronella essential oil**, **lemongrass essential oil, peppermint essential oil, and vanillin** (not imitation vanilla)

Mix all ingredients and place in a travel-size glass spray bottle (the oils can eat away plastic). Store in the refrigerator when not in use. This is a safe and effective formula for everyone including children, unless you have a sensitivity to lemongrass. Other essential oils that are safe for children include catnip and lavender, and these can also be added to your mixture if desired. Babies, children under two years of age, and pregnant people in their first trimester should not use this mix due to risk of ingestion. Essential oils are not safe for many pets, so should not be used on or near them.

Bug Bite remedy: Mosquito bites, bee stings and even ant bites are all a part of summertime fun. It's best if you can avoid them altogether with a natural bug repellent but if they catch you unprepared there are several remedies that should provide relief. Sometimes the remedy depends on what you have on hand. A cool damp green tea bag placed on a bite will relieve itch and inflammation. If you are prone to scratching a bite in your sleep you can place a piece of scotch tape over it until morning. I always keep a bottle of aloe vera gel in my refrigerator in case of burns but it is also good for bug bites. Rubbing a basil leaf on a bite stops the itching. Mixing activated charcoal with a little coconut oil and putting it on a bandage, then applying that to the bite gives relief from the itch and pain of insect bites. Applying witch hazel, tea tree oil, or honey will stop the itch or sting. A paste made from baking soda is said to neutralize bee venom, the same is true of apple cider vinegar.

I can personally attest to the baking soda remedy. It came in handy when I found myself with more than thirty yellow jacket stings. I was using an electric hedge trimmer when I upset an underground yellow jacket nest and they swarmed in an all out attack, apparently instigated by the motor vibrations of the trimmer. The baking soda was the quickest thing I could get my hands on after I managed to get most of the angry beasts off my body. I was in so much pain I literally just poured some baking soda in a container, added some water, mixed it with my bite covered hand and started slapping it on all over my body. By the time I had covered the welts that were forming from head to toe, I realized that the baking soda mixture was all over the floor of the bathroom. That was more than fine because by then it had relieved the pain and I was able to wipe up the bathroom floor which the baking soda mixture left sparkling clean.

Menstrual products: Believe it or not tampons and pads are regulated as "medical devices" and are therefore not required to disclose their ingredients in the packaging.[102] Nearly all of the cotton grown in the U.S. is genetically modified so when this cotton is used in menstrual products it gives pesticide residue direct access to the bloodstream.[103] Since these "medical devices" are used on an exceptionally sensitive and absorbent area of a person's body, they might be interested in knowing what is in said product. Mystery fragrances, dioxins, toxic preservatives, BPA, synthetic fibers, petrochemicals, and high levels of pesticides are just the beginning.[104] It is no wonder that in 2014, House Representative Carolyn Maloney introduced legislation requiring research into the potential health risks of menstrual products, including cervical, ovarian, and breast cancers. Unfortunately, it failed to pass. I would suggest you choose 100% organic cotton, hemp, or bamboo menstrual products. Brands such as Sustain, Natracare, and Seventh Generation are usually available in the health food stores or in the health section of most grocery stores as well as online. There are also reusable menstrual cups made from natural, nontoxic material that are easy to use and good for active lifestyles. They can be worn for up to 12 hours a day, and when it becomes full it can be emptied in the toilet, washed, and re-inserted. These cups usually last about two years. Other nontoxic options include reusable cloth pads and period panties. All of these options are not only better for you but also for the environment, since 12 billion pads and 7 million tampons make their way to U.S. landfills each year.[105]

Vapor Rub*:* Who doesn't have memories of having mentholated ointment rubbed on your chest as a child when you had a cold? We all survived, so how bad can it be? It starts with a petroleum base, which is the first problem, and also contains turpentine oil which, when inhaled, can damage the lungs—and let's face it, that's what you do with these products. Next, we have synthetic camphor, which can cause seizures and should not be confused with the white camphor essential oil.[106] Then, of course, there's added synthetic fragrance, which if you have read any of this book, you know to be very toxic. *Vapor rub alternative:*

- 4 tbsp **coconut oil**
- 1 tbsp **beeswax**
- 10 drops **eucalyptus oil**
- 10 drops **peppermint oil**

Melt coconut oil and beeswax in a double boiler.

Remove from pot, add oils and mix.

Store in a small, labelled, glass jar.

Extra-strength vapor rub:

- 5 tbsp any **oil base**, such as almond for a liquid version, or 4 tbsp **coconut oil** plus 1 tbsp **beeswax**, melted in a double boiler, for a salve version
- 10 drops **eucalyptus essential oil**

- 10 drops **white camphor essential oil**

- A pinch of **menthol crystals** (look for menthol crystals processed from mint plant essential oil, not the synthetic version)

Combine oils and menthol crystals until the crystals are completely dissolved. This mixture is also very good for sore muscles. Note that adding large amounts of menthol to a product can cause skin irritation. Only a small amount is necessary for beneficial results.

An old family remedy to keep you from coughing at night is to rub some on the soles of your feet and cover them with socks before going to bed. When you wake up you will have had a better night sleep and your feet will be nice and soft. One theory as to why this works is because the menthol in the vapor rub dilates the blood vessels in the feet, causing reflexes that soothe the cough, although no one knows for sure. Another theory is that simply breathing in the fumes applied to your feet acts in the same way as applying it to your chest or nose as a decongestant.

As for myself, I use the liquid version daily on my feet after I shower. I found that due to spending long hours on my feet daily, they were becoming calloused. My heels were starting to crack and my feet ached by the end of the day. I rub a small amount into my feet and by the end of the day my feet feel great and look like they've had a pedicure.

Nasal Spray: As with many pharmaceutical or over-the-counter drugs, the side effects of store-bought nasal spray can often be worse than the condition they are treating. Whether from allergies or cold and flu season, an inexpensive bottle of plain **saline** nasal spray will help relieve nasal congestion without potential the side effects of a formulated nasal spray.

The advantage of plain saline nasal spray is that it is readily available, portable, and can be used by people of any age. However, another alternative to nasal congestion is the neti pot. It has been successfully used for centuries to remove allergens, microorganisms, and bacteria from the nasal canal. The process involves the complete irrigation of the nasal canal and can take some practice but may prove to be effective for people in relieving allergies or cold symptoms.[107] There are some very good tutorials on the internet that show detailed instructions on how to properly use a neti pot in the most effective manner. It is important that the water used in the neti pot be distilled or sterilized by boiling then cooled to the proper temperature, warm not hot, as regular tap water may contain impurities. Overall, it is best to try and keep the process as sterile as possible. It should not be used by children, who could potentially choke if done incorrectly.

Antihistamines: Antihistamines have their place when you are having a severe allergic reaction and need immediate help. They can be very effective, however they are not without side effects including drowsiness, nausea, and hyperactivity. If you are taking antihistamines as a way to deal with seasonal pollen allergies, there is a natural solution that might help you: **honey**. Eating local raw honey is a nontoxic way to inoculate yourself to the effects of the pollen in your specific area. The important components of this treatment are that the honey be from a local source thereby providing you protection from the local pollen and that it be raw so that it is still active. You will need to take approximately two teaspoons daily for about three weeks to build the necessary resistance to avoid allergic reactions caused by the pollen.[108] It is best if you can start this regimen early in the season to get a jump on the allergies. It is also important to remember that the honey must be raw so adding it to very hot tea could potentially destroy the benefits. If you cook or heat the honey in any way, it is no longer raw. A recent medical study found that patients who used the local raw honey along with their normal antihistamine used 50% less medication and had better control of their symptoms. It was also noted that those who used the honey as a pretreatment to pollen seasonal allergies had even better outcomes. The study was small in scope, 61 people total, and only looked at reactions to birch tree pollen, however the treatment seems promising.[109] It should be noted that honey should not be given to children under one year of age due to the risk of botulism. Another strategy to relieve symptoms is to eat more onions, especially **raw onions**. Onions contain quercetin that will help your body to control histamine as well as open up your airways making it easier to breathe.[110] The bottom line with allergies of all sorts is that the less toxins that are in your body, the easier it is for your body to handle potential allergens. This is because your liver, being the body's filtering mechanism, can become over taxed dealing with all that modern living throws its way in the form of chemical additives, environmental pollutants, medications, and alcohol. It becomes so overloaded that it cannot efficiently deal with the overactive immune system response created by allergies.[111] Detoxifying and strengthening your liver is a key factor in dealing with allergies. Allopathic medicine often treats allergies by suppressing immune response to allergies, and while this might bring relief of symptoms, it does not address or fix the problem and it adds to the toxic overload which helped to create it in the first place.[112]

Epsom salts and detox baths: Sometimes toxins are unavoidable. Medical tests and procedures such as PET scans and x-rays are all examples of sources of heavy metals or radioactive material you will want to rid your body of, and many people have occupations which expose them to toxins in the air or by direct contact. A great way to remove some of these toxins from your body is a detox bath using Epsom salts.[113] Epsom salt is not a salt but actually magnesium sulfate, a naturally occurring pure mineral compound. The name comes from a saline spring in Epsom, England. Magnesium helps to improve muscle and nerve function, reduces inflammation and improves blood flow and oxygenation throughout the body, while sulfates are important for healthy joints, skin, and help to rid the body of toxins.[114, 115] Adding coconut oil and baking soda to your bath can make the detoxification process even more efficient. It is best to soak for about 40 minutes since you need about 20 minutes to remove toxins, and the second 20 minutes for your body to absorb the minerals in the bath water. Add approximately two cups of epsom salts to a standard size tub under running water to help it dissolve. If desired you can also add one cup of baking soda to warm water. Adding in a 1/2 cup of coconut oil or olive oil is also very good for the skin. Adding any oils to your bath water can make it very slippery and care should be taken when getting in and out of the tub. On a personal note I know several people who, after using hair dyes, have flu-like symptoms that quickly subside after taking an epsom salt, baking soda bath, or using a sauna. Along with these benefits, if you have had a stressful or strenuous day and just want to relax and help prevent the middle of the night leg cramps it can be very beneficial to soak in a detox bath with a few drops of lavender essential oil about a half an hour before bed.

Shower filter: To have the fewest chemicals in your water when showering, you will want to look for a three-stage filtration process for your shower—a micron sediment pre-filter, a Kinetic Degradation Fluxion (KDF) water filter, and a high-grade carbon water filter, as this filters chlorine, disinfection byproducts, and many other contaminants. They are relatively inexpensive, usually starting around $20 and will need to be replaced every six months or so depending on how often they are used. Replacement filters are around $10 . The filters are fairly easy to install, I would suggest a roll of plumbers tape, also called teflon tape (under $2), to avoid any leaking around the filter.

Remove the shower head from the pipe, apply the plumbers tape to the threads on the pipe, screw on the filter, then turn on the water to flush the filter until the water is clean. This will usually take a minute or two, depending on the filter. Now you can reattach your shower head to the end of the filter and enjoy. As an added bonus, now that the shower water is clean, you could hang a sprig of eucalyptus to the pipe of the shower head. The heat and moisture from the water will release the antimicrobial properties of the eucalyptus into the air, providing a host of benefits from easing congestion to making the whole bathroom smell fresh. It is important to ensure that you are using fresh, unaltered, natural eucalyptus leaves and replace them every few months. If you have difficulty finding a local source they are available on many online retail providers.[116]

Vinyl shower curtains: An easy way to reduce the amount of plastic, PVC, and off-gassing in your home is by replacing your vinyl shower curtains. Rather than using older vinyl shower curtains, consider these alternatives:

- Non-PVC vinyl shower curtains

- Organic hemp shower curtains: they resist mildew, dry quickly, are antibacterial, machine washable, and are available online.

- Organic cotton or cotton blend shower curtains: they are a little less pricey than a hemp curtain while also being mildew resistant, machine washable, and available in a wide variety of colors and patterns.

Products Used in the Bathroom and Where to Buy Them

When making your own personal products for the bathroom, it is important to start with pure, quality ingredients and not synthetic substitutes. Organic is always best when available. Here are a few common products you might need and where to get them.

Activated charcoal is inexpensive and available at most drug stores, any vitamin supplier, or online. The source is important for this product. I have found organic, coconut-derived activated charcoal to be the most effective. All of these products are usually available in the "Natural" section of most grocery stores and health stores. Note: as mentioned earlier activated charcoal can interfere with certain medications if ingested.

Organic coconut oil in glass jars are available at Trader Joes and most grocery stores. You can also find affordable liquid vitamin E, jojoba oil, and tea tree oil at Trader Joes, and they have the best non-sale price on Dr. Bronner's bar and castile soap that I have found so far.

The **essential oils** mentioned in this book are never meant to be used by themselves but instead used in small amounts mixed with carrier oils. You should never use essential oils internally, on open wounds or on porous membranes. Essential oils last for a long time, most are good up to ten years if stored in a dark bottle and out of direct sunlight. They are antibacterial, antifungal, and antiviral, making them perfect to add to any homemade cleaning products. True essential oils, especially organic versions, can be expensive due to the fact it takes large amounts of plant matter to produce a small amount of oil, fortunately very little oil is needed for most applications. When purchasing oils it is important to check the label to make sure that they are 100% pure, organic, wildcrafted or unsprayed, have been GC/MS

(Gas Chromatography/Mass Spectrometry) tested, show the botanical name, plant part, country of origin, distillation date, and/or expiration date. Watch for terms such as "therapeutic grade" or "clinical grade" since these terms are not standardized and can be defined as whatever the supplier deems reasonable.[117] A good quality supplier is usually proud of their products and is happy to supply any MSDS (Material Safety Data Sheets) you may request. Some of the best to keep on hand are lemon, grapefruit, eucalyptus, tea tree, rosemary, thyme, and lavender. They are easily absorbed into the skin and do not accumulate in the body over time, so they are perfect to add to personal care products intended to heal, soften, and rejuvenate. Do not apply undiluted essential oils directly to your skin—always use a carrier oil—and never apply them to mucus membranes or take them internally, as this can be very harmful to your health.

- **Orange essential oil** is effective for nourishing dry, irritated, and acne-prone skin.

- **Lemongrass oil** has antiseptic, astringent, and anti-inflammatory properties so when added to shampoos, conditioners, soaps, lotions, and deodorants it can help your skin. The oil also sterilizes your pores, serves as a natural toner, and strengthens skin tissues. In addition, it is said to reduce pain and soothe muscles.

- **Myrtle oil** is antimicrobial, astringent, antiseptic, anti-inflammatory, an expectorant, a decongestant, and deodorizer. In personal care products, it can be used to treat oily skin and, when added to acne skin care products, it makes a good addition to homemade deodorant, and can be included in wound care salves.[118] As a bug repellant, it is known to ward off mosquitoes and other insects. Due to its high tannin content, the herb itself can also be used as a base to treat hemorrhoids.[119] Myrtle oil is often diffused to aid in mental and emotional health, as it is said to relieve nervousness and stress and may help with depression, tension, and insomnia.[120]

Because homemade products do not contain a heavy load of preservatives, they may not last as long as their conventional counterparts, this can be remedied by making smaller batches, or adding **vitamin E** to your formula and storing them in a cool place. It is always best to store your products in glass bottles whenever possible and be sure to label them appropriately. Homemade products can be temperature sensitive. Those containing coconut oil will be more solid when cold and prone to melting when warm. Beeswax and shea butter tend to be a little more temperature stable but can also be affected by extreme temperatures.

Bedroom

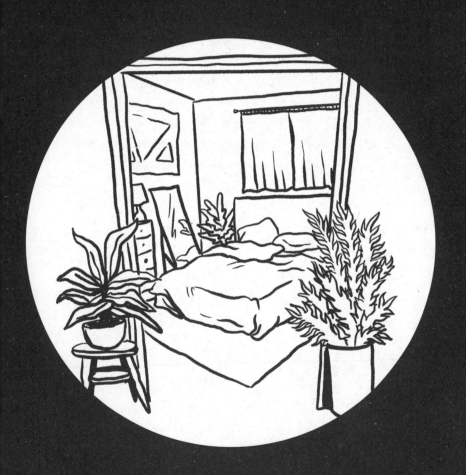

*T*he bedroom is usually one of the safer rooms for toxins, which is good, considering most of us spend about a third of our time in this room. As mentioned in the living room chapter, choosing low or non VOC paints and nontoxic flooring options will be a big help with bedroom air quality. On top of that, proper lighting and air purifying plants are especially important in the bedroom, so let's start there.

Lighting

It is important in any bedroom to create an environment conducive to providing peaceful sleeping conditions. Proper lighting can help to establish healthy sleep cycles, so it is best to avoid LED and CFL lights, as they emit more blue light waves that suppress melatonin production in the brain.[121] Melatonin is a hormone naturally made by your body and is often referred to as the sleep hormone because of its role in developing proper circadian rhythms—your body's wake/sleep cycle. Melatonin levels in your body rise as it becomes dark, allowing you to relax, and reduces dopamine levels, a hormone that helps you stay awake.[122] There are other sources of blue light which can interfere with melatonin production such as computers, laptops, LED televisions, alarm clocks, and of course cell phones. It is best to avoid all blue light sources at least two hours before going to bed, and at the very least keep them out of the bedroom. A better choice for bedroom lighting are incandescent bulbs. For those still having difficulty sleeping, red spectrum bulbs may be the answer. Red spectrum lights, like those used in photo developing rooms, have been found to provide additional health benefits, including improved sleep quality.[123] Red spectrum bulbs also provide for an interesting bedroom atmosphere. The lighting section of the living room chapter offers additional resources for apps available for computers and cell phones to help offset blue lighting on these devices.

Plants

Not only do plants help to provide clean, purified air that is an important part of promoting a healthy sleeping environment, having the right plants can produce relaxing fragrances that may improve your sleeping conditions. Here are a few of the best plants to keep in the bedroom.

- *Valerian*: An herb used in supplements to aid with sleep. A recent study found that the plant itself could help people with insomnia. Participants in the study who inhaled the plant's scent slept longer and deeper.[124]

- *Lavender*: With its sleep-inducing scent, lavender has been shown to have a calming and relaxing effect.[125]

- *Aloe Vera*: Besides being one of the top air purifying plants, it's a great source of fresh aloe vera gel, which is good for soothing burns and other hot spots on your skin.

- *Jasmine*: Not only is jasmine very pretty, it also produces a scent shown in studies to reduce anxiety and improve sleep quality.[126]

Mattresses

Just as with living room furniture, mattresses typically contain highly toxic flame retardants, and there are a variety of other chemicals used in mattress construction that should be avoided for a healthier night's sleep. **Polyurethane foam** and **memory foam** are petroleum-based, and additional chemicals used in the production of these foams, such as Propylene oxide and TDI, have been shown to be carcinogenic.[127] As the foam breaks down, it may release these toxic chemicals into the air, which you in turn can breathe in as you sleep. **Vinyl** is an inexpensive way to make mattresses waterproof. The chemicals used to make vinyl can trigger asthma and allergies,[128] cause genital defects,[129] and alter child behavior.[130] This is why it is so frustrating that vinyl is commonly found in baby mattresses.[131] **Synthetic Latex** is made from two petroleum based compounds, styrene[132] and butadiene.[133, 134] Both of these are VOC's and potentially carcinogenic.

The good news about mattresses is that there is a long list of non toxic mattress makers available online, but there are a few things to keep in mind. Look for full disclosure of materials used in making the mattress, just because it says natural or organic doesn't exclude the use of chemicals or synthetics. When shopping, look for **100% natural latex**, as some manufacturers will use a blend of *mostly* synthetic latex with a small amount of natural latex added and market it as "natural latex." Look for "GOTS" and "GOLS" certification, the Global Organic Textile Standards and Global Organic Latex Standards. Here are a couple to get you started: Naturepedic and Soaringheart.

These websites also provide safe bedding alternatives. The choices you make for laundering your bedding can also impact your health; safe alternatives are available in the laundry section of this book.

Laundry Room

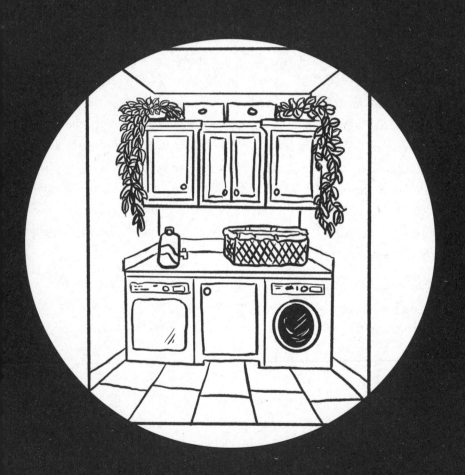

Your clothes are often considered a reflection of the person inside of them. And I'm not talking about designer labels. Clean, unstained, and maybe even nice smelling clothing will always make a good impression. But depending on how this is achieved your good impression might actually be a very toxic one, and the decisions you make when cleaning your laundry can potentially affect not only you but the planet as a whole.

Synthetic Clothing

Not only is the clothing industry known to be one of the most polluting industries on the planet, but the chemicals used in the manufacturing of synthetic, potentially allergenic fabrics like latex, spandex and Lycra are also a huge part of the problem.[135] The dyes used can cause skin rashes, formaldehyde resins used to reduce wrinkling and mildew have been linked to eczema, and nonylphenol ethoxylate (NOE) is an endocrine disrupting surfactant used in clothing manufacturing. When you wash your clothes, these chemicals are released into the local water supplies, and the water treatment facilities are not always able to remove them.[136] Some of the more common chemicals found in clothing include glyphosate, PFCs used to create stain-repellent and water-resistant fabrics, carcinogenic highly toxic heavy metals used in the dyes, and let's not forget about the brominated flame retardants which are known carcinogenic neurotoxic endocrine disruptors, as explored in previous chapters. China and Indonesia have hundreds of clothing factories and as a result some of the most polluted rivers in the world.[137]

Every piece of clothing made from synthetic material produces microfibers that, when washed, shed tiny pieces of non-degradable plastic into the wastewater systems and eventually the oceans of the world.[138] From there they enter the food chain and end up in the fish we eat.[139] The repercussions to marine life and human health is as yet unknown, but are currently being studied.[140]

Maybe you only wear 100% cotton clothing? Unfortunately, unless it specifically states that it is organically grown cotton it will most likely be GMO grown cotton. Beyond just the heavy use of pesticides and herbicides, GMO cotton takes a heavy toll on local water supplies, since the cotton used to make just one T-shirt can take hundreds of liters of water.[141]

There are some clothing lines committed to providing less toxic clothing, and may even show independent lab tests to prove their claims. Look for natural, 100% organic cotton, hemp, or bamboo when making your clothing purchases. They are kinder to the environment and to you.

Beware of labels that say "sustainable cotton" or use the word "blending" instead of "100% organic cotton." Many times, these contain GMO cotton along with the organic cotton. If it has a label that reads "made with organic" it must contain a minimum of 70% certified organic fiber. Also watch for a Global Organic Textile Standards, or GOTS, seal. This means it must contain a minimum of 95% certified organic fibers. GOTS certified textiles are free of pesticides, formaldehyde, chlorine bleaches, heavy metals, and other chemicals that may be harmful to humans and the environment.

Another alternative is vintage clothing, as it creates less waste and most older clothes are less toxic. This is due to the fact that they often do not contain the modern chemicals such as those used to fight stains and wrinkles, for waterproofing, and flame retardants. But be sure to clean them well before wearing to remove any mold or bacteria that may have collected over the years.

Detergent

For most people, your body is covered in clothing almost 24 hours a day. If those clothes contain toxic residue from the cleaning process, those chemicals can be absorbed into your skin, or even inhaled into your lungs. The toxic list of chemicals that can make up commonly found detergents reads like an unpronounceable encyclopedia and if I was to try to list all of the ones that should be avoided, it would fill a chapter. A few are Aziridine, Homopolymer, Ethoxylated, and 1,4-dioxane.[142] It's likely you have seen these chemicals listed as ingredients in personal care products as well, and might think that they must be safe if they are used in those. But if you have read the previous chapters, you know that nothing could be further from the truth. If you choose to purchase your detergent, read the label and look for what it *doesn't* have, like "no bleach," "phosphate free," and "biodegradable." Make sure any fragrance listed is from a non-synthetic, essential oil source. A safe alternative to regular detergent is soap nuts, also called soap berries, a berry shell that grows on the soapberry trees in the Himalayas. They are organic, environmentally-friendly, and have been successfully used for thousands of years. Each tree will provide nuts for about 90 years all the while offsetting greenhouse gases in the process. A good option for people with sensitive skin, they are known to be used to treat skin ailments in some parts of the world and are safe and easy to use for all types of clothes, even silk and diapers. They are also good for use in high efficiency, front loading, or normal washing machines, not to mention there is no soapy residue going into the waterways. Basically, you place about 4 or 5 nuts in a reusable muslin bag and throw it in with the clothes. The clothes can be washed in any temperature and when the washer is finished you simply remove the bag along with the clothes and hang dry it until the next load. Soap nuts are activated by hot water, so if you only use cold water to wash your laundry you will want to place the muslin bag of nuts in a glass of boiling water for a few minutes before adding the bag to your laundry. Soapnuts contain saponin which when added to warm water and agitated creates a soapy lather that removes dirt from the fibers in your clothing. They do not need to be removed during the rinse cycle as they will act as a fabric softener as well. You can use soapnuts to make other household cleaners by boiling ten to twelve nuts in about a quart of water for around fifteen minutes, let the solution cool, add a few drops of your favorite essential oil, and place in a bottle for use in washing dishes or a spray bottle to clean floors and counters. They will last for about ten loads. Once they start to become soft and grey you can throw the 100% biodegradable nuts into the compost bin. Note: it may take several washings to remove the old detergent from your clothing.

Fabric Softener and Dryer Sheets

These products coat your clothes with a layer of chemicals which can then be readily absorbed into your body. The most common unpronounceable chemicals used in these products are called "QACs," short for quaternary ammonium compounds. These chemicals are referred to as "asthmagens" as they can cause asthma to develop in otherwise healthy people.[143, 144] In addition to QAC's, these products also contain synthetic fragrances, often so strong that those who use them can be identified in a crowd of people by the familiar permeating smell. Even being near a home when the dryer containing these products is running will fill the air with the scent, as well as pollute it with these allergy promoting and asthma producing toxins.[145] This is another area where our grandparents had the right idea: hanging your clothes outside to dry will freshen, soften, and even brighten them as well as eliminating all static cling. It is environmentally friendly and lowers your electric bill. This may be more of a challenge depending where you live. Here in the Pacific Northwest's winter months, I have hung sheets out in the sun only to find it raining on them ten minutes later, so be sure to check the weather. When it's not possible, there are safe alternatives that can be used instead. The easiest way to reduce static cling is to roll up a sheet of aluminum foil and throw it in the dryer with clothes; it can be reused several times. A more environmentally friendly alternative would be 100% wool balls as they provide many benefits. They will help your laundry dry faster, greatly reduce static cling, aid in removing wrinkles, help to fluff the fibers which softens the fabrics, and they last for years. You can add a few drops of your favorite essential oil to the wool balls if you prefer scented fabrics. Below is another quick and easy way is to make your own **scented fabric softener**:

- Tie a 100% cotton washcloth into a knot and pour a small amount of white vinegar (about 1/8th of a cup) into the center.

- Add a couple drops of your favorite essential oil like lavender (which has antibacterial properties as well as producing a relaxing fragrance) around the knot.

- Throw it in with the clothes.

Once dry the clothes will be soft, very lightly scented, and mostly static free.

Whiteners

Optical brighteners used to make your clothes seem cleaner actually leave a coating of microscopic fluorescent particles which create an optical illusion that tricks the eye into thinking that the clothes are clean and bright.[146, 147] These optical brighteners are often made from benzene and can be very toxic. When they rub off onto the skin they can create a rash, irritation, or allergic reaction, which can be worsened by sunlight.[148] Chlorine bleach, another whitening product, is also highly toxic, especially if combined with other cleaners known to cause respiratory problems like asthma.[149, 150]

The Alternatives: Add a cup of hydrogen peroxide to the washer with your whites, let them soak in a tub full of water for about an hour, then finish washing as usual. Adding a cup of lemon juice is also a good choice and can be used in place of the hydrogen peroxide. Or, soak clothes in a mixture of one part white vinegar and six parts water overnight, then wash as usual in the morning. Lastly, one of the best natural whiteners is using the ultraviolet rays of sunlight by simply hanging the clothes outside on a sunny day.

Stain Removers

The laundry list of toxic chemicals in stain removers can irritate your skin, eyes, and respiratory system. Add to that allergens, asthmagens, and possible carcinogens, it's not something you want in contact with your body. Once these chemicals are added to the wash water they enter the water system and environment, causing even more damage. The solution is simple: a quick mix of borax, castile soap, and hydrogen peroxide. I mix about one part of each in a labeled glass container and keep it above the washer. I find a toothbrush works best for application. It works great on any stain including oil, grass, wine, and even blood. Just apply a small amount of the solution onto the stain, brush it in with the toothbrush and wash as normal. If there is any doubt as to color safety on the clothing to be treated, you can omit the hydrogen peroxide and use only the borax and castile soap.

Dry Cleaning

I am not sure where the expression "dry cleaning" came from, as it's not dry at all: garments are placed in liquid solvents to remove the oils and dirt. The toxic culprit in this cleaning process is called "perc," short for perchloroethylene. Perc sounds much nicer, and you would never suspect that it is categorized as a toxic air pollutant by the EPA, linked with cancer and other serious health effects. In fact, the air in and around dry cleaners has higher contamination levels of perc.[150] No surprise there, but what is surprising is that they found the highest levels in low-income and minority neighborhoods, possibly due to poor ventilation systems in the buildings.[151] If you must use a dry cleaner, look for an eco-friendly one that uses a non-perc solvent or, even better, pressurized CO_2. Just make sure to do your homework because technically perc is considered "organic" as a carbon-based solvent. And in consideration of the environment and yourself, don't forget to bring your garment in with a reusable garment bag, so your clothes don't end up in plastic.

A better alternative to dry cleaning would be to steam your garment, which kills the bacteria that cause odors, or use a microfiber brush to gently brush any oils or soil from your clothes, which is very effective for wool suits. You can also hand-wash your clothes in a little borax and castile soap, then line dry, unless you are washing silk or wool, then you should reshape to air dry by laying the piece of clothing on a flat rack in the shape you want it to dry in. Never squeeze or wring out delicate clothes, they may be blotted with a towel to remove excess water.

Dry cleaned fabrics should be aired out in an *unpopulated* area, like the garage, before bringing them into the bedroom, to avoid the off-gassing of chemicals into your home.[152]

Kitchen

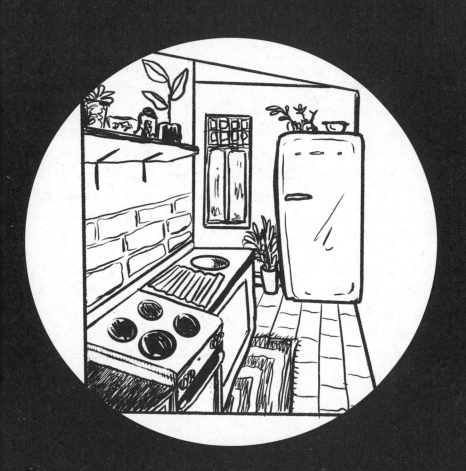

*T*he kitchen is a landmine for toxic chemicals from many sources: the cleaners used, the appliances for preparing food, and even the food itself. Modern conveniences like microwaves and coffee makers have made life easier and less time consuming, but they come at a cost. Even water, one of the most basic elements used in the kitchen, can be a source of toxins. Let's start with that.

Water

It is recommended that a person consume half their body weight in fluid ounces per day to be adequately hydrated. This means a 150-pound person would need to drink 75 ounces of water or comparable fluids per day for healthy hydration.[153] That being said, it would be a good idea to make sure that while endeavoring to stay hydrated you are not poisoning yourself in the process. This may be harder than you think. According to research from the nonprofit research organization, Environmental Working Group, tap water contains over 250 chemicals and pollutants. Among them are pesticides, herbicides, heavy metals, and the ever-present endocrine disrupters.[154] Most of the US water supply also contains industrial chemicals such as polyfluoroalkyl and perfluoroalkyl (PFASs). These are known carcinogens. Even more frightening, several pharmaceuticals including antibiotics, anticonvulsants, sex hormones and mood stabilizers have been discovered in public drinking water supplies.[155, 156, 157] At this point, many public water supplies in our country are polluted due to various factors.[158] These include toxic runoff from industrial factories, improper disposal of medications, and agricultural runoff from Concentrated Animal Feeding Operations (CAFOs).[159] The tap water from these public water supplies is also used to make commercial beverages like soda, juice, and coffee as well as being the source for 60% of bottled water.[160] Research conducted on bottled water at the State University in New York found microplastic contamination in 93% of the samples. The tests on more than 250 bottles from eleven brands showed contamination with plastic, including polypropylene, nylon, and polyethylene terephthalate.[161]

If you live in the US, you may be one of the 170 million who drink radioactive tap water. We rely on government agencies to protect us from harmful elements like radioactive tap water. However, at times, even the government testing conducted for the purpose of ensuring safe environmental standards has been found to be skewed. For example, Kathleen Hartnett White, a former chair of the Texas Commission on Environmental Quality, admitted in a 2011 interview with KHOU-TV to knowledge that the commission falsified data as it pertained to excessive radiation levels to make them appear to be within safe levels, as correcting the problem would have been too costly.[162]

According to EWG tests from 2010–2015, more than 22,000 utilities serving over 170 million people in all 50 states reported radium in their water.[163]

Even well water is no longer exempt from manmade chemicals since the development of fracking. This is a process of drilling down into the earth and injecting highly toxic chemicals at high pressure into the ground in an effort to release natural gas deposits. These chemicals can eventually end up in the ground water. No one even knows what is contained in the highly secretive concoction used by the industry for this practice.[164]

Water filters

Now that you know what is in the water you'll need to know how to remove it. To do this you will need the appropriate water filter. There are many filters available on the market. The least expensive and most readily available are taste and odor filters: they will do little to reduce the toxins in your water, but it will taste better.

A better choice would be a good quality NSF (National Sanitation Foundation) certified granular carbon and carbon block filter. They are available in both countertop and under the counter models. They remove contaminants and should be able to provide a list of exactly what they remove, verified by lab testing of their products.

There are also reverse osmosis filters, which work by forcing tap water through a semipermeable membrane and additional filters to remove impurities from water, which will also work to filter out chemicals like fluoride. We purchased a system for less than $200 after finding fluoride, and then had the water tested again after installing the filter and no traces were detected.

On a personal note, I had the experience of hiking for two days in the Goat Rocks Wilderness area in Washington to the glacier at the top and along the way I drank the clearest, sweetest tasting water from the springs that the same glacier created. If you ever have the opportunity to experience fresh, glacial mountain spring water right from the source, you will never forget the taste or energizing feeling that it imparts. It usually requires a substantial hike, but is well worth the effort.

Microwave Ovens

Many health conscious people have already given up their microwave ovens, but few actually know why they're considered to be unhealthy. Microwave ovens work by causing dielectric heating, or heating the water molecules in the food, causing them to vibrate at extremely high frequencies billions of times per second. The structures of those molecules are ripped apart and forcefully deformed. This process damages the nutritional value of the foods heated.[163] Cooking food by any method damages the nutritional value to some degree, however, due to the nature of microwave cooking, the damage goes beyond just having less nutrition. If the food you are cooking is packaged in plastic, the toxic chemicals can leach out into the food as it is cooked.[164]

Cookware

Cookware is something you use every day, often several times a day. Most food contains sodium in some amount, which acts as an acid in the cookware, causing metals to leach out into the food. So, if your cookware is leaching metals or chemicals into your food, then you are eating those metals and chemicals several times *a day*.[165] Some of the worst offenders are non-stick cookware, which begin leaching chemicals into your food after being heated for just five minutes and will fill the air with toxic chemicals if overheated. This is of particular concern if you have pet birds, as fumes from an overheated non stick pan will kill a bird in a very short period of time. Aluminum cookware and inexpensive Stainless-Steel cookware leach aluminum, chromium, and nickel.[166, 167] Recent research has linked the accumulation of aluminium in the brain to such diseases as Alzheimer's and Parkinson's disease.[168] Lastly, avoid "Green" recycled cookware, since there is no way to know where they obtained these recycled metals, or what they were originally used for.

There are safer alternatives, but they are not without their own issues. There are cheap cast iron products that use synthetic seasoning, for example, but the best are the old, true, well-seasoned **cast iron** your grandparents cooked with. Cast iron will leach iron in small amounts which can be instrumental in treating or preventing anemia.[169, 170] For most people, cast iron is a good alternative but for those with genetic factors involving excessive iron levels, there are other options.

Ceramic cookware should be safe, however some of these products have been found to contain lead and cadmium when imported from other countries.[171] There are several brands available on the internet, many with certification of purity from lead and other toxic substances. Coated ceramic non-stick cookware is supposed to be safe, as long as there are no scratches, chips, or other sorts of damage to the pan. **Tempered glass** cookware, on the other hand, is a safer cooking option.

Titanium Cookware is a good non toxic alternative that is strong and lightweight, but can be very expensive. If you are considering titanium cookware make sure it does not have a toxic nonstick coating.

Stainless Steel Cookware can be a good choice if you choose pans made from high quality 18/8 stainless steel made in America. These numbers indicate the composition of chromium to nickel used to make the stainless steel. I purchased a set of T304 (a rating equivalent to 18/8) **surgical stainless steel** cookware set 34 years ago and I am still using it to this day. The downside is that while it is guaranteed for life, the initial cost is very high.

Coffee makers

A staple in most households, this appliance gets the morning off to a good start, especially if you are using fair trade, organic coffee. Coffee is an acidic beverage, and between that and the hot water needed to brew the coffee, you may be getting more than you bargained for. The plastic from most coffee makers, whether BPA free or not, shed the chemicals used to create the plastic into your daily brew, and thus into you.[172] If you have read any of the previous chapters you already know what plastic can do to your body, so you get the idea. Single use and typical automatic coffee makers are susceptible to mold and mildew growth which, besides making the coffee taste bitter, can pose health risks when consumed. It is therefore very important to clean the coffee maker often, white vinegar and water work very well, then dry the reachable areas with a cloth and leave it open when not in use.

If you are trying to avoid plastics in your coffee, look for one made of glass or stainless steel, or at the very least find one with no plastic parts that come into contact with the coffee. The old fashioned stainless-steel or glass percolators are generally safe as long as they are not made with aluminum parts. A french press is *usually* plastic free, as well as some of the modern all-glass pour-over coffee pots that feature a wooden collar and natural paper filter. As more manufacturers are becoming aware of consumer concerns over plastic, more and more are developing stainless steel alternatives with food grade silicone water transport hoses. These are typically available online, so do some research on current options before making your purchase.

Flatware

The expression "born with a silver spoon in your mouth" came from the idea that the wealthy families used silver utensils while the poor family's utensils were made of lead, tin, or pewter. This may have kept those using the silver spoons healthier, due to the germ fighting properties of silver, whereas the poor may have been ingesting small amounts of lead from the flatware with their daily meals. Silverware has many advantages over flatware, as it has antibacterial properties and can even kill microorganisms.[173] This is the reason silver was placed in containers of milk or water before refrigeration was invented, as it prevented bacteria from forming.[174] You can still purchase silverware or silver-plated utensils, but they are not inexpensive. I found a set of 1847 Rogers Brothers silver-plated utensils in an antique store at a very reasonable price. However, when buying antiques, it is important to make sure that the silver-plating has not worn off, as you cannot be sure what is underneath. There are many other safe options available, for example bamboo, as long as it is not coated with anything, and good quality stainless steel (18/8) utensils. If all else fails, you can always use untreated chopsticks. The one to avoid is plastic; it's bad for you as well as the environment.

Plates and cups

Anyone with children knows the value of plastic or melamine dishware. What they might not know is that the toxic chemicals from these plates, bowls, and cups can easily end up in their food. There are two main types of plastic in dinnerware: melamine and polypropylene. Both are hazardous to human health, with children being even more vulnerable to the effects.[175] A study done in Taiwan showed individuals who consumed hot soup from melamine bowls had absorbed various amounts of melamine into their body, as it was found excreted it in their urine. The amount of melamine varied depending on the brand of tableware used.[176] Many factors can affect the leaching of plastic or melamine, such as if the food is hot when it makes contact with the tableware. When microwaved in such a container, a greater amount is present in the food.[177]

A safer alternative would be to use ceramic tableware in general and uncoated bamboo as an unbreakable option for small children. This is also true for bowls used to feed your pets.

Food containers

The container you use to store your food or leftovers may not seem important but, if it is in plastic wrap or a plastic container it can release toxic chemicals into the food. Where do I start? Cling wrap is made from polyvinyl chloride (PVC), which leeches harmful substances that cause a myriad of detrimental health effects.[178] It is nearly impossible to avoid plastic these days, as most grocery stores wrap all fresh meats, and even some produce, with the stuff. You may be one of the fortunate few shoppers that can order meat from a butcher, but most of the paper they use to wrap the meat, is coated in a film of plastic as well. At this point the most you can do as a consumer is to minimize your exposure by removing products from their plastic containers and transferring them to glass as soon as you get them home. When shopping, look for condiments or beverages already in glass. When possible, take your own glass containers to the store when purchasing bulk items and meat, if you have a butcher. I know that it isn't convenient to carry heavy glass containers around, but then neither are the effects of years of exposure to plastic and the toxins associated with it. I am old enough to remember when everything came in glass containers, and yes they were heavy, yes they broke if you dropped them, but they were recyclable and nontoxic. They didn't end up in the oceans or as toxic chemicals in our bodies. As for other alternatives to plastic wrap, there are several companies making nontoxic food wrap from 100% organic cotton treated with beeswax. These wraps are usually reusable for long periods of time, depending on how you care for them, and when they do wear out, are biodegradable. They are also a great solution for children's lunches where glass containers are more susceptible to breaking. There are more and more biodegradable container options being introduced to the market, however it is still important to make sure they are nontoxic. Stainless steel, bamboo, food grade silicone, and glass storage containers are readily available just about anywhere. If you are looking for storage options for freezing food you can use glass mason or ball jars, but be sure to only fill three quarters full.

You can also wash and reuse milk and ice cream cartons for sauces and soups, and for short term freezing, you can use unbleached butcher paper.

Cleaners

If you look under the kitchen sink of most homes you will probably see a myriad of spray bottles that promise to clean and disinfect every conceivable surface in your kitchen. While they all promise to make the job easier, they do not tell you about the chemical consequences of using them. They usually have warning labels that include instructions such as using in a well-ventilated area, rinsing off completely, keeping out of reach of children, and sometimes even include the poison control phone number just in case you didn't read the first few warnings. But there are many natural alternatives for general cleaning without the chemical consequences.

A good **castile soap** is great for washing dishes, mopping floors, and cleaning just about any surface in your kitchen. A bottle of castile soap under your kitchen counter will replace about five of those other, toxic spray bottles.

Hydrogen peroxide is a great disinfectant for cutting boards, children's eating surfaces, and even meat-contaminated countertop surfaces. It is very inexpensive and available in a spray bottle.

Baking soda works great as a scrub and can be combined with a little borax for problem areas. For stubborn counter or sink stains you can sprinkle baking soda on the problem area then spray some hydrogen peroxide over that. Then simply wipe it off.

There are a number of nontoxic cleaning products available online or in health food stores, but as mentioned before, it is important to read the labels.

Avoid synthetic fragrances or words you cannot pronounce. And, when possible, try making your own cleaners with the recipes in this chapter.

Oven cleaner

One of the top three most toxic cleaners on the market, oven cleaners usually receive failing marks for safety when rated by the Environmental Working Group. The other two most toxic are toilet bowl and drain cleaners.[179] Even the Poison Help Hotline states "Oven cleaner poisoning can cause symptoms in many parts of the body" such as difficulty breathing, severe pain, intestinal burns, vomiting, and more.[180] I would have to add another chapter to list all of the toxins that can be found in these products. Instead, let me suggest an alternative:

Mix the following in a spray bottle:

- ¼ cup **castile soap**
- ½ cup **lemon juice**
- 1 cup **white vinegar**
- 1 ¼ cup of **warm water**

Be sure to remove any baked-on food residue with a spatula before starting, then spray the inside of the stove generously. Baking soda may be sprinkled on top of stubborn stains that have been sprayed. Allow the mixture to remain for 30–45 minutes then rinse off. Application of elbow grease may be required for some areas.

Ant Repellant

Kitchens are magnets for pesky ants, and there are many commercial products that promise to rid your home of them, some will even continue to kill them for months after the initial application. It's not that you are going to eat the bait yourself of course, but having them in and around your home adds to the toxic load that you, your children, and your pets are exposed to on a daily basis. There are many safe alternatives that are easy and inexpensive to make. Here are a few techniques I recommend.

Cinnamon

Cinnamon acts as a natural ant repellant when used in high enough doses. Here's what you'll need:

- ½ tsp cinnamon essential oil
- 1 cup water
- Cotton balls or cloth

Mix cinnamon essential oil with water.

Soak a cotton ball or a cloth in the mixture.

Wipe your counters and other areas where you spot ants.

Repeat once a day until the ants disappear.

You can also leave a few drops of straight cinnamon essential oil near doors and windows for extra protection.

Vinegar

Another natural mix that repels ants.

What you'll need:

- Apple Cider Vinegar
- Water
- Lemon essential oil, peppermint oil or cinnamon oil
- Spray bottle

Mix equal parts of apple cider vinegar and water in a spray bottle.

Add a few drops of essential oil of choice or combination thereof.

Shake well before each use.

Spray wherever you see ants.

Repeat daily until ants are gone.

Borax

If you find that repelling them is not enough then you can use this recipe to eliminate them. You may notice more activity around the bait as it will attract them and they will take it back to their nest and share it. The borax mixed in with the bait will ultimately kill the entire colony.

What you'll need:

- 2 tbsp peanut butter
- 2 tbsp sugar
- 1 tsp borax
- 1 tsp water

Mix all ingredients together and place in a shallow container.

Seal with lid and poke a few holes through the top and the sides, so only ants can get in and out.

Place the bait container in the area where you see the ants.

Make sure to keep this away from your pets.

Food

The food we eat today has changed dramatically from what our great grandparents ate. As a child I once saw a television show where a man who appeared to be a scientist in a lab coat brought out a beautiful lemon meringue pie produced entirely of chemicals. There wasn't a lemon or egg in it, even the crust was comprised of chemical ingredients. The scientist proudly explained what chemicals were used to produce each of the pies components. At the time, this was seen as progress. Back in the 1950's the food industry was making tremendous strides, producing foods that were fast and convenient to prepare. No one even considered how these chemicals would affect their bodies.

Unless the food you are eating is truly organic and properly washed, it is most likely heavily contaminated with pesticide and herbicide residue. To make matters worse, the regulations concerning these standards are changing daily, and often for the worse. As of 2019, to be sold or labeled as organically produced agricultural products according to the USDA they, "must not be produced on land on which any prohibited substances, including synthetic chemicals, have been applied during the 3 years immediately preceding the harvest."[181] If produce is labeled as transitional it means that no prohibited substances are being used but that it has not been a full 3 years preceding the harvest. Certain chemicals and pesticides are allowed in organic farming. The label does not guarantee that the food will be completely free of toxins.[182] The FDA allows the word natural to include additives like high fructose corn syrup, artificial preservatives like potassium sorbate, and sodium benzoate (which are made from industrial chemicals), hexane, and genetically modified ingredients, just to name a few.[183] Truth in labeling can be deceiving: I read a label the other day that said "non-GMO coconut oil" in big bold lettering displayed right on the front of the label, so while the coconut oil was non-GMO (there are no GMO coconuts grown at this point in time), the other ingredients listed on the label that were commonly GMO sourced were not explicitly identified as non-GMO. There is a lot of controversy surrounding the health effects of modern day agricultural practices, and there many terms used to describe what is being done to our food (e.g. GE or genetically engineered; GMO, genetically modified organisms; GEC, gene-edited crop; and mutagenesis, which is changing the genetic information of an organism).

GMOs: You may have heard the argument that farmers have been using genetic engineering techniques for centuries. In fact they did, to some extent. It started when they began saving the seeds from the hardiest plants for replanting. Often the seeds that produced the best flavor or highest yield were saved so that the line would continue. The next step was the introduction of cross pollination. This was often done in closely related species in hopes that it would produce the desired traits of extra flavor or disease resistance in the next generation. Many of the familiar fruits and vegetables we find on our table were born from processes like these including carrots, oranges, broccoli, and kale, among others. However, the techniques used were not always successful and the results were often unpredictable. Then came hybridization, which was done by breeding different plants many times over until they obtained a stable strain that could be cross pollinated to grow plants with more predictable results. However, the seeds produced from these hybrids were not the same as the plants they came from, so the farmers had to purchase new seeds each year. In the early 1980s, the first genetically modified organisms were created by inserting genetic material from one organism into the DNA of another. A large percentage of GMO crops were developed so that certain unnamable seed companies could use massive quantities of their herbicide on farms without harming the crops. It was a win-win situation for them because farmers were forced to buy their herbicide tolerant seeds and use their proprietary herbicide every year in order to stay viable. Without getting into the politics of whether or not seed producers are trying to take control of the world's food supply, as some have asserted, let's look at what the food produced by these different methods do to our bodies. I'll use corn as an example, since it has been around a very long time and used by many ancient civilizations. Corn in its natural, unaltered state contains the enzymes needed by your body to make it exponentially more bioavailable, meaning your body can easily digest most of the nutrients available in this corn.[184] This is why it was highly prized and considered a staple in many cultures. Once the corn has been hybridized it loses some of those enzymes in the breeding process and it is less bioavailable but still nutritious and nontoxic. Once it is genetically modified with the DNA of soil bacteria and doused with glyphosate, it is no longer the nutritious staple of the past and is better suited for corn ethanol than corn on the cob.[185] Far from the healthy staple that sustained the people of many cultures for centuries, corn has become an ingredient to be avoided in all its forms, from high fructose corn syrup to tortilla chips.

How about wheat, another staple of many diets? Though not genetically modified yet, it has been so manipulated and changed over the last few decades that your body may not recognize wheat molecules as food and attacks it in an effort to protect you. This may account for the modern epidemic of gluten intolerance among the population.[186] Another problem with (non organic) wheat is the use of glyphosate as an herbicide and as a desiccant to allow the wheat to dry sufficiently to be harvested. Washington State University (WSU) researchers have found a variety of diseases and other health problems in the second- and third-generation offspring of rats exposed to glyphosate.[187] Many doctors advise their patients to avoid GMOs in their diets, citing pregnant people, babies, and children as being "the most likely to be adversely affected by the toxins and other dietary problems" related to GM foods.[188] In all fairness, there are some scientists (usually the ones that work for the seed companies) that will tell you that GMOs are safe, nutritious, and going to save the world. But I am old enough to remember what scientists said about tobacco and, like Big Tobacco, these companies spend millions of dollars to fight labeling laws and convince the public of their good intentions. Many would contend that further research is needed to satisfy the public that GMOs are safe, however research on industrial GM crops are subject to patent-law limitations that may limit the scope of a researcher's ability.[189] This could also have the potential for a conflict of interest or even the suppression of information.

Navigating the grocery aisles in an effort to provide your family with healthy food can be a challenging process these days. A simple rule of thumb is to avoid the center aisles where the most processed foods can be found. Things in boxes, bags, and cans. Beyond that, read the label, if you see artificial colors, additives, preservatives, and BPA coated canned items, put the item back on the shelf. Purchase organic produce to avoid pesticide residue and GM food that your body may not recognize, or that may produce allergic reactions or digestive issues.

The following section covers a few of the staple items you may encounter daily, with information to help you in making decisions to purchase the healthiest options.

Canola oil: If you are a health conscience, label-reading consumer, you probably see canola oil listed as an ingredient in most products these days. It is usually one of the first ingredients listed on the label of healthy snacks or condiments, since it is inexpensive to use. This is the reason companies often use it to replace the more expensive olive oil.

There have not been any long-term studies done on the health effects of canola oil—for better or for worse. However, preliminary research indicates that it may have a negative effect on heart health and even memory.[190] A better alternative is a high-quality organic olive oil, which has been studied and proven to have health benefits, including lowering cholesterol, reducing the possibility of developing type-2 diabetes, and aiding in heart health.[191]

Sugar: If you are reading the labels of the products you are buying in an effort to keep yourself and your family healthy, you may know how difficult it can be to identify the ingredients on the label. Sugar may be listed multiple times under any of the 61 names used to describe it, so the product may contain large amounts of sweeteners even though they are not necessarily listed first in the ingredients. Some of the more common ones that you may recognize are high fructose corn syrup, maltose, glucose, sucrose, and dextrose. Some not so common include muscovado, demerara, castor, panocha, sorghum, and treacle, to name a few you may not be familiar with.Taking that into account, it is easy to see how the average American consumes 71.14 grams, or seventeen teaspoons of sugar daily, even though the recommended amount is 25 grams, or six teaspoons.[192] But is it toxic? Many believe it is a major contributing factor in many of the diseases currently affecting humanity. It contains no nutrition, causes tooth decay, overloads the liver, can cause insulin resistance, weakens the immune system, and causes the release of dopamine in the reward center of the brain, making it highly addictive.[193, 194] Studies show that drinking two sodas or eating the equivalent of 100 grams of sugar will suppress your immune system function for up to five hours.[195]

While we know that sugar is toxic and addictive, it is also nearly impossible to avoid. One morning while visiting an elementary school I saw a group of children having breakfast before classes started. They were eating yogurt which contained nearly 30 grams of sugar, as well as artificial food dyes that may cause hyperactivity.[196] I could only imagine how difficult it was going to be for them to sit and concentrate on the studies to come. According to the cafeteria supervisor this was the only breakfast some of those children would get and, even though she agreed that the nutritional value was minimal due to the additives, it was what the district provided, as it was low cost. To be fair the children had other options to choose from such as (previously frozen) french toast strips made from white bread presumably dipped in egg and coated in a sugary coating with syrup, cereal also containing high amounts of sugar, artificial colors, and, as we have now become aware, even glyphosate, sugary juice, and a piece of fruit. Surely it is better that these children have something to eat than go hungry but in a perfect world (or one that cared about their children) these little growing bodies would be provided with healthy nutritious food devoid of toxic chemicals regardless of their ability to pay for it. Even the CDC (Center for Disease Control) recognizes the correlation between healthy eating and higher test scores.

High glucose corn syrup is a highly processed sweetener used in most processed foods and beverages, as it is inexpensive and highly addictive. A study at the University of Princeton found that high fructose corn syrup (HFCS) caused obesity and substantial increases in triglyceride levels, both known risk factors in humans for heart disease, cancer, and diabetes.[197] Further research also shows how fructose promotes pancreatic cancer growth and that it should be aggressively avoided when trying to prevent or treat pancreatic cancer, the pancreas being the organ responsible for insulin production.[198] Even though HFCS can be labeled as natural in ingredient lists and you may have heard that your body cannot tell the difference between it and regular cane sugar, neither of these claims are accurate.[199] At the risk of getting all scientific on you, cane sugar consists of two molecules, glucose and fructose, in equal amounts, bound tightly together. The enzymes in your digestive tract break it down into its component parts and absorb them into the body. HFCS is also glucose and fructose but not in equal amounts, and in an unbound form that is not broken down by enzymes but rapidly absorbed into your bloodstream. The fructose goes directly to your liver, increasing cholesterol and triglycerides, and can cause a condition known as "fatty liver." The glucose triggers a spike in your insulin which can lead to increased probability of an overactive appetite, weight gain, diabetes, heart disease, and cancer.[200, 201]

The Alternatives: **Raw honey** is a superfood that contains enzymes, antioxidants, vitamins, minerals, and promotes a healthy digestive tract. As an added benefit, if the honey is local, it can help relieve pollen allergies. Unfortunately these benefits only refer to raw honey, once it is pasteurized (or cooked) it loses many of these properties.[202] Additionally, honey should not be given to children under one year of age due to the possibility of containing botulism spores.

It is best to look for raw, organic honey, and, believe it or not, not all honey sold in stores is real honey. To increase their profits some honey providers add other, less expensive, sugar sources to a small amount of real honey and sell it at the higher price of real honey. Look for "100% Pure" honey, which is thick, has a slight aroma of flowers, and caramelizes quickly when heated. Your best option is to buy it from a beekeeper or farm directly.

Stevia is another alternative, and has been used for hundreds of years in South America. It is 100–300 times sweeter than sugar so it takes very little and is available in many forms like liquid, tablets, powder, and even in packets for on-the-go.[203] It has no calories or carbohydrates and helps to support healthy blood sugar levels and weight loss.[204] Note: Make sure the source of stevia you are buying is plant based rather than chemically made and that it contains no chemical additives. You can grow organic stevia yourself, dry the leaves, and crush them into a powder using a mortar and pestle, and add them to anything you would like to sweeten. However, powdered leaf stevia is inexpensive to purchase and less labor intensive.

Organic Coconut sugar has a low glycemic index and is rich in minerals which include zinc, potassium, magnesium, calcium, copper, polyphenolic compounds, vitamin C, and other antioxidants. Because it has a lower level of fructose than normal table sugar, coconut sugar is less likely to contribute to fat deposition. The unique form of fiber found in coconut sugar, inulin, has been linked to lowering overall cholesterol levels in the body. It resembles light brown sugar and can be used in baking or added to your morning coffee.[205] Note: while coconut sugar is a better alternative to regular sugar, it is still a sweetener and should be used sparingly.

Organic maple syrup is a good source of minerals and antioxidants. Studies have shown that it can inhibit cancerous colon cell growth when applied directly to cultured cells.[206] Maple sugar can provide your body with antioxidants, which fight the effects of free radicals and help to prevent cancer.[207] It has a low glycemic index and contains abscisic acid. Abscisic acid is a natural defense in controlling diabetes because it has the potential to encourage the release of insulin through the pancreatic cells.[208]

Maple syrup comes in Grades AA, A, B, C and D. Grade D is the darkest of the five and contains more of the beneficial antioxidants than the lighter grades.

Organic Cane Sugar is considered "unrefined sugars." Because it is less processed, it has a sweeter taste and still contains some of the nutrients present in cane juice.

Salt: Salt is necessary for a healthy body. There is salt in every cell in our body, keeping all the processes in proper balance.[209] You may have heard that too much salt is bad for you but the truth is that not all salt is created equal, and even a small amount of the wrong kind is bad for you. Table salt is the most common and widely used. It is a highly processed, manufactured form of sodium chloride stripped of all of its minerals, with added ferrocyanide, aluminum, anti-caking agents, and iodine. Table salt raises your blood pressure by retaining water in your bloodstream, putting a strain on your heart.[210] Packaged foods, processed foods, and most fast foods contain very high amounts of this type of salt. **Kosher salt** on the other hand, is harvested from evaporated seawater and is not as processed as table salt. It does not usually contain the added iodine and anti-caking agents.[211]

Sea salt also comes from evaporated sea water but is a smaller grain that Kosher salt, but still contains the minerals present in the area it was harvested. A concern with sea salt is that it may contain microplastics. Microplastics are tiny pieces of plastic, smaller than 5 millimeters, that are formed when larger pieces of plastic start to break down. In a study from 2018 published in the peer-reviewed Environmental Science & Technology scientific journal, more than 60% of salt sold across the world contain microplastics, with the highest levels found in sea salt.[212] I particularly enjoy celtic sea salt. It's harvested in Brittany, Fance near the Celtic Sea using a 2000 year old method said to preserve the nutritional benefits and therapeutic qualities. This salt is slightly grey in color and remains moist to the touch regardless of how it is stored. It has a very nice taste and a little goes a long way so you will need less. **Himalayan pink salt** is said to be the purest salt in the world and is harvested in the salt mines of the Himalayas. These crystallized sea beds that make up the mines are over 200 million years old, which is what gives this salt a perfect crystalline structure. It contains 84 natural minerals and elements found in the human body and does not contain the impurities and environmental pollutants now present in our modern sea salt. Besides being an asset to your health, Himalayan salt has a wonderful taste.[213]

White flour: You might think that in recent years we have made great strides in improving the nutrition of white flour, but instead we have made great strides in the *processing* of white flour. We start with wheat that has been genetically engineered, possibly causing digestive problems in certain people. Since 1996 there has been a noticeable increase in the number of reported instances of celiacs disease.[214] This wheat is then treated with fungicides, pesticides, and insecticides, then bleached using any number of the 60 different approved chemicals before removing the bran and six outer layers, which contain 76% of the vitamins and minerals as well as 97% of the fiber. Then we age it with chlorine dioxide and add chalk, alum, ammonium carbonate, and potassium bromate (a category 2B carcinogen[215]). White flour can also contain alloxan to make bread look fresh, which is harmful to the pancreas according to studies and is used to induce diabetes in animal experimentation.[216]

The Alternatives: There are many healthy grains, just keep them organic, whole, and minimally processed. **Whole grain** bread provides fiber and naturally occurring vitamins and protein. **Sprouted grains** contain more protein, less fat, and are easier to digest than whole grain while also containing less gluten. **Amaranth**, a super grain from the Aztecs, is very high in protein, minerals, fiber, and is gluten free. And because of its squalene content, a compound that helps to inhibit cancer, it is considered one of the healthiest grains.[217] There's also **Tibetan barley flour** (Tsampa)[218] which is high in fiber, has been shown to reduce the chances of developing heart disease and diabetes, and is used by hikers to sustain energy levels.

Milk: Milk is an interesting subject in itself. It is not so much that milk is unhealthy, it is what we do to it in the production process that makes it less than an ideal source of nutrients. There are many variables involved, starting with the type of cow providing the milk. There are two types of milk, A1 and A2. The A1 versus A2 factor refers to the different type of casein in raw milk from various breeds of cows. Casein is a milk protein. Put simply, A1 casein milk is hard for humans to digest and causes bloating and gastrointestinal problems. A2 casein does not cause these problems.[219] A2 milk is produced only from cows having two copies of the A2 gene for beta casein. A high percentage of Guernsey and Jersey cows produce A2 milk, whereas most Holstein (the more familiar black and white cows) produce A1. It is a matter of genetics, however, and you can change the genes of any breed to produce A2 milk. New Zealand, Australia, and Africa, where A2 milk is common, are all countries that have known and practiced this for years. Other countries are starting to take note and you can find milk labeled A2 in most major grocery stores. On a side note: all goats' milk is A2 regardless of the breed and is usually very easy to digest. The cow's diet is another factor in determining the nutritional value of the milk produced. 100% grass fed cows produce milk with higher amounts of omega-3[220] and conjugated linoleic acid, also known as CLA. CLA is an important nutrient because of its association with cancer fighting properties.

Besides the type and the diet of the cow, it is also important how the milk is processed. Modern advances led to homogenization, which took care of that pesky cream on the top problem. However, homogenization makes the fat molecules too small to be digested in the stomach so they can be absorbed into the bloodstream and seen as a foreign protein by the body.[221] The body reacts to foreign proteins by producing histamines, then mucus. Then milk is pasteurized, to prevent listeria and other illnesses, which can be life threatening to those with compromised immune systems. Raw milk and raw milk products should be avoided if you are pregnant due to the potential for miscarriage if the milk in tainted. With all that in mind, milk produced from GMO fed, corporate-controlled processing and distribution systems, known as Confined Animal Feeding Operations, or CAFOs, is far from what nature intended, and may not be the healthiest option.

The Alternatives: 100% grass-fed non-homogenized, non-pasteurized milk from Jersey cows in glass containers. It is very important to make sure that the laws in your state allow the purchase of raw milk, and that the provider of the milk be reputable and conscientious. To locate a raw milk source near you can go to the *Real Milk* website at realmilk.com. Remember that any other dairy products such as cheese, ice cream, sour cream, yogurt, etc. should come from organic and 100% grass fed sources as well, to avoid potential toxins. If you cannot purchase raw milk, the next best alternative is non-homogenized, 100% grass fed, organic milk, which is available in most supermarkets. However, grass fed, organic, non-homogenized A2 milk is available at most health food stores.

Eggs: Eggs have oscillated between being demonized and prized throughout the past few decades. They were once thought to contribute to heart disease, then later thought to prevent it. It's hard to know what to believe. Basically, eggs can be good for humans and, like sugar, salt, and red meat, all things in moderation is the key to good health. Several studies have shown that eating two to three eggs a day lower bad LDL cholesterol and raise the good,[222, 223] and eggs contain many vitamins and minerals including choline, which is essential for brain and nerve health.[224] Other nutrients that can be found in eggs include lutein and zeaxanthin, both of which are abundant in the yolk and vital to eye heath and may slow macular degeneration.[225] Tryptophan and tyrosine amino acids are also potent mood enhancers.[226, 227] Not all eggs are created equal, and free range, pasture raised, organic eggs are far superior in quality to the eggs of factory raised caged hens fed GMO diets.[228] They typically contain more than a third more vitamin

A, a third less cholesterol, and two times more omega-3 fatty acids.[229] The best way to eat these eggs, to retain as much nutrition as possible, is raw. The less an egg is cooked the more nutrition it retains, so much so that the antioxidant properties of an egg are greatly reduced when it is fried or boiled.[230] The cholesterol in the yolk of an egg can be oxidized by high temperatures, especially if it has been scrambled.[231] You may be concerned about the risk of salmonella, and rightly so. It helps to avoid eating eggs obtained from chickens raised in factory farms, where living conditions can prove very unsanitary.[232] "You are what you eat" applies to chicken's eggs as well, depending on where they are raised, as conventional factory farms feed their chickens inexpensive GMO feed. The resulting eggs have pale yellow yolks. Pastured and free range chickens, having access to insects and a wider range of vegetation, produce eggs with orange yolks and the darker the yolk the higher nutrition content.[233] Any hormones or toxins in the bloodstream of the hen can end up in the eggs and that includes the stress hormones of hens in overcrowded and stressful conditions.[234] This is another example of how considering the source of your food can affect the health and welfare of not only the animal, but also those who consume the food produced by them. We are lucky to be able to have four hens, even though we live in the city. They are free range, organically fed, and eat the bugs in our garden. They provide beautiful eggs with nearly orange yolks which I add raw to our morning smoothie. As a way of giving back to the chickens for their kind contribution, I leave a little of the smoothie in the blender and add the egg shells and banana peel, then re-blend it up and serve it to the chickens to help replenish any vitamins they may need to make more eggs. It may seem downright disturbing to feed them their own eggs, but it is a widely accepted practice and it must be helping, as they are more than seven years old and still laying eggs almost daily.

Meat: Science has proven that the meat from animals raised in Confined Animal Feeding Operations, or CAFOs, and fed GMO feed contains high levels of antibiotics while also having less overall nutritional value than the meat of 100% grass fed animals.[235, 236] In 2011 nearly 30 million pounds of antibiotics were sold to meat and poultry producers. This practice is contributing to the problem of antibiotic-resistant disease from which at least 23,000 Americans die every year.[237, 238] Even if we *don't* take the health of the animals and the very land they are raised on into account, this is an unhealthy and unsustainable way to produce meat. If everyone would commit to reducing their meat consumption to just three times a week, and purchased sustainably raised meat each of those three times, we could effectively eliminate Confined Animal Feeding Operations, or CAFOs, completely. CAFOs are a leading cause of greenhouse gases, they contaminate drinking water, and the animal waste stored in open ponds is often sprayed on food crops as fertilizer.[239] That waste can contain pathogens, heavy metals, and antibiotic-resistant bacteria. Besides its potential effect on the food crops themselves, it enters the environment causing numerous health issues in humans.[240] Children near the farms have higher asthma risks and there are respiratory issues for adults as well as headaches, nausea, weakness, and chest tightness.[241] The health and welfare of animals in CAFOs and factory farms is tragic. They spend their entire lives in extremely cramped conditions living on concrete in their own excrement, with no access to pasture, fresh air, or natural light. They are routinely fed antibiotics and GMO feed. At the end of their tragic life they are subjected to the industrial slaughterhouse, which takes inhumanity to a whole new level. They are treated not as living beings but as a commodity. Their tails, ears or, in the case of chickens' beaks, are often cut off. They are then forced to be constantly medicated due to unsanitary living conditions. Illness and infections are part of the process and are ignored until they are "processed" for meat. It is no wonder why our meat is high in levels of stress hormones.[245] Even the farms themselves are a source of danger for the communities neighboring them. The potential public health impacts associated with these farms include airborne MRSA organisms and soft skin infections.[246, 247] The nutrition and health benefits of meat from animals raised on grass and not grain is astounding. Cattle, pigs, and poultry raised on their natural pasture and grass-based diets produce meat that is lower in total fat and calories, higher in good fats like Omega 3's, higher in concentrated antioxidants such as vitamins E, C and beta-carotene, and that has increased levels of other disease-fighting substances.[248, 249] Grass-fed meat has 2–4 times more omega-3 fatty acids and 3–5 times greater amounts of another good fat called Conjugated Linoleic Acid (CLA) than CAFO-raised meat.[250] CLA is a polyunsaturated fatty acid that's been shown to help fight cancer, discourage weight gain, and build muscle.[251] So, limiting your meat consumption to three times a week with grass-fed, humanely raised, organic meat is not only better for you, but it is better for the animals and better for our environment.

Produce: Organic is always best. In an effort to stretch our food budget I always look for organic produce that is on sale and plan our meals around them. Occasionally if organic is not an option for a particular item needed, there is a solution. Literally, a solution: mix one teaspoon of baking soda in 2 cups of water and soak your produce for 15 minutes, then rinse and enjoy. According to a study using apples this method removed more pesticides in 2 minutes than using a mixture of bleach and water.[252] This method is also very effective for soft produce such as berries or leafy greens that may otherwise be difficult to wash. All produce should be washed in this manner before use for a number of reasons, one being that the organic label doesn't mean completely free of pesticides. In fact, it means no synthetic chemicals were used but may have been treated with natural and organic pesticides, which are developed completely from plant and herb components. It should also be noted that pesticides are able to penetrate the skin of produce and must be peeled when possible to be avoided. When you can not buy organic it is good to know which produce poses the greatest risk and which are the safest. EWG provides a list on their website of what they refer to as the dirty dozen, this is a list of fruits and vegetables that contained the highest concentrations of pesticides. These include: strawberries, spinach, kale, nectarines, apples, grapes, peaches, cherries, pears, tomatoes, celery, and potatoes. Kale and spinach had more pesticides by weight than any other crop. So whenever possible it is best to go with organic when purchasing those, especially when children are involved. There is also a list of what they refer to as the clean fifteen which included: avocados, sweet corn, pineapples, frozen sweet peas, onions, papayas, eggplants, asparagus, kiwis, cabbages, cauliflower, cantaloupe, broccoli, mushrooms, and honeydew melons. Few pesticides were found on these foods, in fact their tests showed only 6% of the samples had residue of two or more pesticides and more than 70% of those listed had no pesticide residues.[253] Farmers markets are also a great source for safe, less expensive produce as most grow their produce organically but have not gone through the expensive certification process to have it labeled as such. A lot of the vendors at these markets usually have signage stating their growing practices or are happy to inform anyone asking about them.

Detox with Beets

Organic beets are a great example of healthy, beneficial produce. Amazing detoxifiers, they can improve athletic performance, help fight inflammation, lower blood pressure, lower your risk for heart failure and stroke, help combat cancer, and improve brain function.[254] They are also great for pregnancy because they are high in the B vitamin folate, which has been shown to alleviate morning sickness, particularly fermented beets.[255] Beets are high in sugar, so if you need to avoid sugar, it is best to use fermented beets as this removes nearly all of the sugar during fermentation.[256] Beet juice is another option, but fermenting your beets gives you all the benefits of raw beets plus you get beneficial bacteria and enzymes, and the fermentation process makes all of the nutrients in beets more bioavailable. Fermented beets have been used to boost immune function, cleanse blood, combat fatigue, and treat kidney stones, chemical sensitivities, allergies, and digestive problems.[257] Since beets are so great at detoxifying, be careful about overdoing it in the beginning as this could result in an overload of released toxins, producing bloating, constipation, or even flu-like symptoms.[258] If you are juicing, it is best to start out with 1 ounce per day, gradually increasing the amount to an 8-ounce glass per day. If you're highly toxic, meaning you are an alcoholic, abuse drugs, live on nothing but fast food, or considered medically toxic from chemo, etc., you may need to start out with as little as a tablespoon. The liver has to "filter" and process the toxins your body is trying to get rid of, so flooding an already overworked liver would be counterproductive. I always recommend buying organic beets or growing your own from heirloom beet seeds.

Nursery

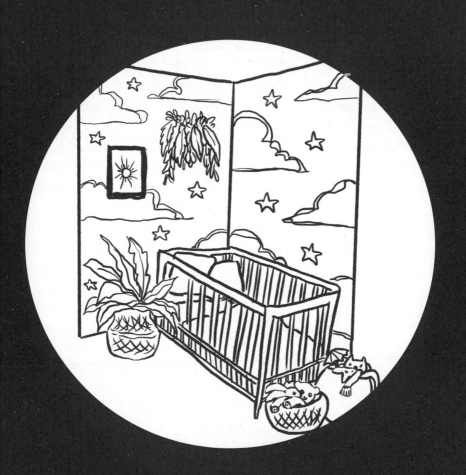

*B*abies and young children are the most susceptible to the toxins we encounter in our everyday lives. Unfortunately, even the personal care products designed for use on babies and children contain known carcinogens and chemicals that can affect brain development and cause liver and kidney damage.[259] Toxic chemicals in this room can come from many sources such as carpeting, paint, food, plastic bottles, bedding, fire retardants, and even medications and pharmaceuticals. It is no wonder that today's children have far more allergies, asthma, and illnesses than those of a generation ago. In 2009, the Environmental Working Group commissioned a laboratory test conducted on the umbilical cord blood of U.S. newborns and their findings proved that US infants are contaminated with BPA in the womb. More tests on these same samples were conducted by five laboratories in the US, Canada, and Europe. They found up to 232 toxic chemicals in the cord blood samples, including flame retardants, synthetic fragrances, pesticides, and chemicals used to make non-stick cookware, textiles, food packaging, and other consumer products.[260] It is so important, now more than ever, to provide your baby with the least toxic environment possible, before and after birth, to give them the best start in life.

Baby Body Products

It goes without saying that you want the safest products for your baby. If you are buying a store-bought baby personal care product, be sure to read the label, and remember, if you wouldn't eat it don't put it on their delicate skin. Use common sense when using anything on a baby. Natural doesn't mean safe. If it has fragrance, put it back: it is most likely synthetic and your baby doesn't care how it smells (that being said lavender essential oil can have a calming effect on you and the baby). Organic coconut oil makes a great moisturizer, but remember that it takes very little. Cornstarch is a good replacement for talcum powder. For bathtime, Dr. Bronners makes a nice unscented liquid castile soap just for babies that works for the whole body, including use as a shampoo, and is available at most department stores.

Baby Wipes

Baby wipes are admittedly a necessary requirement for any modern parent with a baby that needs changing, but these can be very toxic. Even though they may contain some nice sounding ingredients like castor oil or aloe vera, it's the rest of the ingredients that will get you. Baby wipes typically contain preservatives like Bronopol also known as 2-Bromo-2-nitro-1,3-propanediol. Bronopol contains the following warning: "Harmful in contact with skin, harmful if swallowed, causes skin irritation, may cause respiratory irritation, causes serious eye damage, and is very toxic to aquatic life."[261] Another preservative to avoid is DMDM hydantoin, which releases formaldehyde as it breaks down.[262] There are some safe alternatives on the market but they can be quite expensive. The Environmental Working Group website rates them for safety. A far cheaper alternative would be to make them yourself. You will need:

- A roll of **paper towels**. 100% Bamboo dioxin free paper towels available online are the best choice for health and sustainability. There are also reusable options, however a good quality heavy duty brand of any strong paper towel will work.

- A **large container with a lid**, big enough to house half of the paper towel roll.

- 2 cups of **distilled water**

- 2–4 tbsp **aloe vera**

- 3 tbsp **witch hazel** (non-alcohol)

- 1 tsp **Dr. Bronners** or any castile soap

- a few drops of **vitamin E oil**

First, cut the roll of paper towels in half (I find this is easiest with a long serrated knife) and place it cut side down in the container. Mix all ingredients together and pour over the paper towels, allowing the liquid to be absorbed. Make sure to keep the container tightly closed when you are finished using it so that the wipes do not dry out.

Diapers

Not only are diapers an environmental waste nightmare, they contain unlabeled cancer-causing chemicals much like menstrual products.[263] Toxins found in disposable diapers include dioxins, ethylbenzene, phthalates, toluene, styrene, dipentene, sodium polyacrylate, tributyl-tin, VOC's, synthetic fragrances, and dyes. Any one of these alone can cause anything from skin irritation, damage to the liver, or changes in the genes that promote obesity and cancer, just to name a few.[264] When these chemicals mix together they can also create toxic emissions that may cause respiratory problems.[265] Luckily, there are options available for purchase that are mostly chemical free. One disposable diaper that seems promising is called "Little Toes Baby Diapers." They are made with soft 100% chlorine free bamboo fibers, do not contain dyes, fragrances, or lotions, and are 100% biodegradable. According to the EPA, the estimated generation of disposable diapers in the US in 2015 was 4.3 million tons,[266] and while the jury is still out on how long it takes a disposable diaper to biodegrade, with some saying 500 years, others saying never, it is important to think about the world you want your baby to inherit.

In a perfect world, the best alternative would be organic cotton, hemp, or bamboo reusable cloth diapers washed in soap nuts and dried with lavender essential oils or air dried in the sun. There are many options available for purchase online or you can make your own. There are also free patterns available online as well as sizing suggestions. Using organic sources for your cloth means less chemicals and pesticides next to your baby's skin and a cleaner environment.

Formula

The first years of a baby's life can have a profound effect on their future. What you feed your baby will affect their brain development, teeth, and overall health. With so many parents working or unable to breastfeed, formula is a convenient and often necessary option, and the formula industry rakes in over $8 billion a year and promises to provide your baby with the essential nutrition it needs. Formula has come a long way since it was first patented in 1865 by a chemist who combined cow's milk with wheat flour, malt flour, and potassium bicarbonate. But even as an adopted baby myself, whose first few months were spent ingesting Karo syrup and evaporated milk, I consider myself fortunate that many of the formulas now on the market were not available then. While the mixture that I was fed had little nutritional value, at least it didn't contain the toxins in the formulas that babies have to contend with today. Some common ingredients in baby formulas are as follows:

Soy based formulas, in general, are one cause for concern. Most are from GMO sources and contain pesticide residue, but soy itself contains phytoestrogens which may disrupt thyroid function, sexual development, immune function, and even brain development, though more studies are needed on the topic.[267] Carrageenan is a food additive that comes from seaweed, which doesn't sound bad but it has been labeled as a possible carcinogen and linked to gastrointestinal ulcerations and tumors in mice.[268] DHA and ARA are synthetic fatty acids extracted from algae and fungus using hexane, which are meant to replicate the fatty acids naturally found in breast milk, but the synthetic versions have been found to possibly cause gastrointestinal distress.[269] Then there's sugar. All formulas will contain some form of sugar, just as a mother's milk does. It is necessary to digest the proteins in milk. But not all sugars are created equal. Avoid corn sugars, HFCS, and lactose, which many companies are now using because it more closely mimics human milk. Even organic formulas can contain as much sugar as a can of soda.[270] What can you do to avoid feeding your little one a host of toxic chemicals? First read the label. Organic doesn't equal safe, but it usually means that you are able to avoid GMOs, pesticides, antibiotics, and growth hormones. Many of the ingredients in organic formulas can also be problematic, like the sweetener brown rice syrup that was found to contain six times the EPA's safe level for inorganic arsenic.[271]

The Alternatives: Breast is best! This goes without saying, but breastfeeding is not only good for the baby as the parent receives many benefits that go far beyond just strengthening the parent-child bond. Parents who breastfeed typically lose weight faster after childbirth due to the fact that they burn about 500 extra calories a day building and maintaining a milk supply. Nursing stimulates the uterus to contract and return to normal size. Parents who nurse also experience fewer urinary tract infections, have less chance of anemia, and less risk of postpartum depression.[272] The benefits to the baby are impressive and believed to continue well into adulthood. They start with a stronger immune system, less stomach issues, fewer colds and ear infections, less allergies, and lower rates of sudden infant death syndrome. It can even prove protective against pediatric cancer as several studies have shown a protective association from acute lymphoblastic leukemia in babies who are breastfed until at least six months of age, the most common pediatric cancer in the United States.[273]

As breastfeeding is not always possible, organic European formulas are often the best choice for those who can afford it, the next option being organic US formulas. There is a website that rates products based on heavy metals and contaminants including baby formulas and foods. It is called the "Clean Label Project" and can be accessed at cleanlabelproject.org/product_catagory/formula.

Bottles

So now that you have decided what to feed your baby, you will need a safe container to put it in. Whether feeding breast milk or formula, you want to make sure the bottle is free of toxins that may leach into its contents. While the FDA has banned BPA from baby bottles, some manufacturers have started using bisphenol-S (BPS) instead, which may prove even more harmful.[274] Studies have shown that even the BPA-free plastic bottles are found to leach other harmful estrogenic chemicals.[275]

Glass may very well be the best option to avoid plastics leaching into the liquid. Most are made from thermal, shock-resistant borosilicate glass. They should come with medical grade silicone nipples and are available in various shapes, depending on the baby's needs.

Crib mattress

Choosing the right mattress for your baby is even more important than the one you choose for your own bed. Babies and children are more susceptible to environmental toxins than adults, and your baby will spend a lot of time sleeping on what could be a chemical nightmare. Studies have shown that when babies spend time sleeping on typical crib mattresses they are exposed to elevated concentrations of chemicals released from the mattresses.[276] In fact, a 2015 study at Texas University found that crib mattresses released nearly 30 different types of Volatile Organic Compounds (VOC's) as well as other harmful airborne chemicals.[277] The body heat produced by the baby increased these emissions, which were the strongest in the infant's immediate breathing zone. Besides breathing in the chemicals, an infant's sensitive skin can also absorb certain toxins. Most crib mattresses contain chemical flame retardants, polyurethane foam, and are made with waterproof covers using PVC. These chemical exposures can negatively affect your baby's health and brain development and there is speculation that the toxic gases produced by the cribs could be a major cause of Sudden Infant Death Syndrome (SIDS). New Zealand started a death prevention campaign in

1995 in an effort to reduce SIDS. Their theory was that if a baby breathed or absorbed lethal doses of the toxic mattress chemicals it could potentially shut down the baby's central nervous system, stop the breathing and then heart function. Between 1995 and 2013 at least 235,000 babies participated in the campaign. The test subjects slept on properly wrapped beds to block the chemical gasses from getting to the babies. During that time, no deaths reported for the babies on the wrapped mattresses, while there were 1,020 deaths reported on unwrapped mattresses.[278] Clearly, while more research is needed on the subject, there is definite evidence that toxic gasses in crib mattresses should be avoided. That being said, how do you do that? There are a few things to watch for.

When a mattress says it is organic, it may only be referring to the outer cover and the inside may still contain toxic polyurethane foam. Look for full disclosure of all materials used.

If you decide on a waterproof mattress, make sure to avoid vinyl and PVC, look instead for food grade polyethylene.

Make sure that the flame retardants used in the mattress are not chemical based but that the mattress meets the flammability regulations by using wool, cotton, or natural latex.

The good news is that there are actually many mattresses available (usually online) made from GOTS certified organic cotton, organic wool, 100 % natural latex, and eucalyptus. They have been tested and certified by third party labs such as Greenguard, Standard 100, or Oeko-Tex for chemical emissions so you and your baby can rest assured they are the safest available.

Paint, carpeting, lighting, and clothing have been covered in the preceding chapters—Just remember that when using any of these products in a nursery, it is very important to make sure they are as free of toxins as possible.

Pet Products

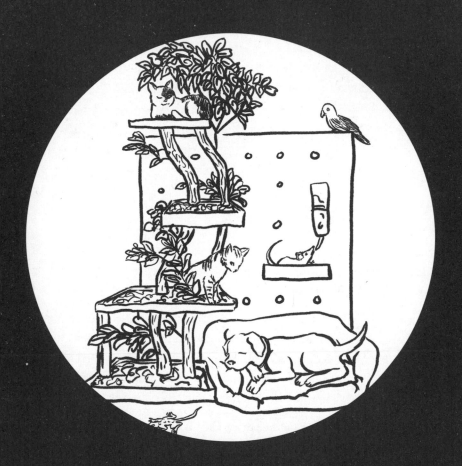

*F*rom service animals to family pets, animals enrich our lives in many ways. Pets have a calming effect on people of all ages and it has been proven that children raised in households with dogs have less allergies and asthma.[279] Other health benefits of owning a pet include decreased blood pressure, cholesterol and triglyceride levels, and increased opportunities for exercise and socialization.[280] I worked as a Vet Technician back in the early 1980's, and things have changed dramatically in the way we treat our pets. Now there are entire animal clinics devoted to cancer treatments, allergies, and heart problems. Over six million dogs and cats are diagnosed with cancer every year, and those are just companion pets, unlike the farm animals that end up in the food chain.[281] Just like humans, what your pet eats, along with the environment they live in, has a profound effect on their quality of life. It is unfortunate that most veterinary schools teach very little on the subject of nutrition. Instead they rely on a handful of major pet food companies to conduct seminars for vet students, and guess what they are teaching them to feed your animals? Your pet is exposed to endocrine disruptors from many areas: plastic food, water bowls, chlorinated water, chemicals used to clean your home and lawn, and even the flame retardants in your furniture and pet bedding. The following chapter covers some of the things you may have never considered that could be impacting your pet's health.

Bedding

Like people, our pets are susceptible to the same toxins in our environment, though it takes less to make them sick as animals are generally smaller and have faster metabolisms than humans. Pet beds made from synthetic materials are sprayed with toxic flame retardants, and your pet can then inhale these chemicals as they off-gas, or even ingest them when they clean themselves. In fact, because they are constantly grooming themselves, cats have been found to have high levels of flame retardant chemicals in their blood.[282] A better alternative would be a pet bed made with organic cotton and silk. Both can help reduce overheating, which can help prevent hot spots and allergies. Another bonus is that dust mites, another allergen, cannot survive in silk. Pet beds made from these materials are available on the internet and, while the price is higher than the synthetic version, they are strong and washable. My favorite so far has been an organic cotton and silk pet bed available on Mercola.com.

Flea Deterrents

Pyrethroids (man-made chemical insecticides) are used in flea sprays, room foggers or bug bombs, and collars to kill fleas, but these chemicals are very dangerous to humans and pets alike. For example, the monthly spot-on treatments to kill fleas may pose many health threats, prompting at least nine class action lawsuits against the makers of these products.[283] Just reading the precautions on these products might make you think twice about using them at all.

The Alternatives: **Diatomaceous earth** is a nontoxic alternative to flea products. It is actually made up of the fossilized remains of tiny aquatic organisms called diatoms, made of silica, which work against fleas by dehydrating them, killing the little buggers. It can be sprinkled in the yard and on your carpet. Let it sit on the carpet several hours before vacuuming. Diatomaceous earth is harmless if consumed but should not be inhaled. You can also apply it directly onto your dog or cats coat, avoiding contact with their eyes and nose as well as your own. For a **nontoxic flea spray**, mix one gallon of vinegar, ½ gallon of water, sixteen ounces of lemon juice, and eight ounces of witch hazel together and place it into a garden sprayer. You can then use it to spray your carpets, furniture, pet bedding, and window sills to get rid of fleas.

To make a **carpet powder**, mix one part Borax to two parts baking soda in a shaker bottle, shake contents over rugs, allow to sit for several hours, then vacuum to deter fleas. It is best to keep pets and children from playing on the carpet until it is vacuumed. Any residue that remains in the carpet after vacuuming will continue to kill fleas.

Dog Baths

There are many safe herbal shampoos to not only clean your dog but also deter fleas. It is best to avoid toxic pyrethroids (synthetic pesticides), so check the label for D-trans allethrin, resmethrin, pyriproxyfen, and s-methoprene. If they are listed, you may want to choose another brand. When bathing your dog, brush them first, protect their ears using a wash rag around their face, and rinse very well to avoid dry skin and itching. If the dog has thick fur you can dilute the shampoo with water before working it into a lather, which will help it get through the fur and make it easier to rinse out. A diluted solution of betadine can be used to help sanitize hot spots or areas that may itch.[284] Foot baths can be beneficial when your dog has walked through grassy areas that may have been treated with chemical herbicides, or in the winter when sidewalks have been treated with chemicals to melt ice.

Spaying and Neutering

First of all, you must know that I am pro-sterilization, it is an important step in preventing overpopulation, which leads to the euthanasia of the unwanted animals. However, the techniques used by most veterinarians remove all the organs that secrete sex hormones, including estrogen, progesterone, and testosterone. That may not seem like a bad thing until you realize that these hormones are needed to provide normal biological functioning throughout the animal's lifetime. Most animals are spayed or neutered by six months of age. That would be the equivalent of a ten year old girl having a hysterectomy and not expecting any side effects. Not having these hormones can affect everything from the brain to the bones, especially in a young animal that is still growing. Once these organs have been removed the animal's body has to try to get these hormones in other ways. The only organ left that can produce sex glands is the adrenal gland, which now has to work overtime to do its normal job and the job of the missing organs. This is the reason these animals often have allergies, shorter life spans, joint problems, and immune system issues. This was proven in a study done by the School of Veterinary Medicine, UC Davis, that found various cancers and joint problems in higher numbers of neutered animals than in intact animals.[285] If you have a pet that is already spayed or neutered using mainstream methods, you can help them by supplementing the adrenal glands, by feeding your animal raw organ meat from grass-fed cows. Raw so that it will contain the enzymes needed for proper digestion, organ meat to help support the overworked adrenal gland, and grass-fed so that the organs which filter out pesticides and other toxins, like the liver, will be clean and healthy for your pet. It should be noted that there are dangers associated with any raw diets or supplementation with raw meats due to possible bacterial contamination. This can be avoided by using any of the many supplements available in pet stores or online for adrenal support. If, however, your pet is still intact and you are considering having them spayed or neutered, consider talking to your vet about alternative sterilization procedures, such as a vasectomy for males and a modified ovary-sparing spay for females, which only removes the uterus.

Pet Food

Pet food may be one of the main culprits in the unhealthy state of most animals today. Typical pet foods today are biologically inappropriate, overly processed, and contain so many toxic ingredients, it is surprising that the animals are doing as well as they are. Food dyes are used in almost all of them, and not so the animals will eat the food but so that the consumers will think it looks more nutritious.

Most commercially produced pet foods use a base of corn, wheat, or rice and many people have only recently begun to realize that feeding carnivores a grain-based diet can cause cancer and creates overweight, diabetic animals. As a result of this, many started producing grain-free diets instead. Unfortunately, these usually contain inappropriate levels of high-glycemic starches or carbs such as legumes that can cause GI inflammation. To add insult to injury the cans containing the pet food also contain either BPA or PVC based coatings (sometimes both) and this includes some of the organic brands as well.[286] The best diet for your pet is a balanced, raw, homemade diet. However, this is very expensive, time consuming, and requires a lot of research to do properly. It can also be dangerous if not done properly and is not recommended for young pets. There are commercially available raw diets that might work for you, and while far more convenient, they are not cheap. However, if they help to avoid costly vet bills and prevent your pet from suffering, they may be well worth the cost. If you do decide to feed your pets a raw diet, be sure to transition them gradually from their dry food diet over time. Another healthy alternative to the dry kibble is a freeze-dried raw diet. Freeze dried diets are not processed at high temperatures so they retain their nutrient content, and they are a convenient and easy way to feed a raw diet: just add water. This is an added bonus if you enjoy camping or traveling with your pets, since freeze dried diets are shelf stable and light-weight to carry. High quality foods are more expensive, but there is a trade off in that pets consume less of the nutrient dense foods, since it doesn't contain the empty calories that leave them hungry for more nutrition, and they are usually healthier as a result. The bottom line when choosing pet food, as with anything else, is that it is important to read the label and avoid as many toxic ingredients as possible in your price range. Note: It is important not to try to feed your pet a raw or cooked homemade diet without the knowledge to do it correctly. It usually ends up being nutritionally unbalanced, causing endocrine abnormalities and organ degeneration. Please refer to the Pet Food section of the "Tried and True" chapter for commercially available sources of raw and freeze dried diets.

Treats

Whether for dogs or cats there are an abundance of treats available on the market these days. It may be difficult to know what is safe for your pets with all of the choices available. As a general guideline, look for treats made from ingredients that are sourced in the US, then try to avoid added sugar (in all its forms), artificial colors, artificial preservatives, chemicals, and grains, especially corn as it is known to be highly allergenic to some pets. You can also create your own treats by starting with a high quality canned food and freezing small, bite-size portions on a cookie sheet with parchment paper. Keep them in an airtight container in the freezer to be given as needed. Another simple treat is to take a sweet potato and slice it thinly, then cook it in the oven on low until it becomes dehydrated and chewy. You can do the same thing with the meat of your choice. You can leave it in strips or cut it up into little training treats. Keep what you are not using in the freezer. Remember, treats should be given in moderation.

Dental Chews

Because conventional diets are so far from natural, pets today often have very poor dental health. There are any number of dental products on the market to combat this problem. While most veterinarians recommend that you never give your pet "cooked" bones as they can splitter and cause digestive problems, some veterinarians have suggested "raw" bones, under constant supervision, to aid in the removal of dental tartar.[287] However, I would suggest talking to your pet's veterinarian before giving them any bones. If you choose dental chews for your pet, it is important to read the label in order to avoid sodium hexametaphosphate (SHMP), a chemical often used to coat these treats. SHMP is a man-made industrial polymer. According to Material Safety Data it is hazardous to humans if swallowed and can cause reactions ranging from vomiting to kidney failure.[288] One of the easiest things I have found has been to slice an inexpensive cut of meat into strips, such as turkey breast, then freeze them. There are no sharp splinters to worry about, no chemicals to make your pet sick, and they are hard enough to clean the teeth. Smaller strips work best for cats. Note: since the meat should be raw, it is best to feed your pet on a mat that can be washed when they have finished.

Pet Dishes

Just as for humans, pet's dishes should be ceramic, glass, or stainless steel, never plastic. They are subject to the same toxic chemicals as humans with the exception that it takes much less to affect them. It is important to keep the dishes clean and free of bacteria by washing them regularly with a nontoxic soap such as Dr. Bronners.

Kitty Litter

The choices are endless when it comes to litter options so it can seem overwhelming: clumping, non-clumping, dust control, odor control, beads, pellets, crystals, scented, unscented, and even biodegradable. There are health implications when using the clumping clay litter, because most contain sodium bentonite which, according to the Material Safety data sheet,[289] contains crystalline silica. When inhaled, this is a group 1 carcinogen that causes irritation of the skin, nose, throat, and airway passages, and can lead to permanent lung damage. Bad for you and your cat. Corn based kitty litters, besides being from GMO sources, can be contaminated with aflatoxin, which are poisonous carcinogens that are produced by certain molds activated by moisture like urine and have been linked to liver failure. Even the biodegradable litters have their drawbacks; recycled paper can include chemicals and inks, wheat pellets can contain the herbicide glyphosate, walnut hulls will not break down if your pets ingest them, and grass pellets typically contain pesticides.[290]

The Alternatives: There are some organic corn varieties, as well as some wood litters, that are free of chemicals and fragrances. Some pet owners make their own litter by using chicken feed and adding a little baking soda. If using any form of corn based litter, it should be changed often to avoid any aflatoxin risks. Sand is another inexpensive alternative and baking soda can be added to this as well. Wheat based litters are another option.

Choosing a Veterinarian for Your Pet

So much has changed since the days when I was a veterinary technician in the late 70's and early 80's. When your pet needed care you took them to the local vet and, if they were unable to handle the problem, they might have consulted one of the very few specialists available in the field. Unlike today with Veterinarian Specialists in Allergies, Oncology, Heart, Orthopedics, and even Holistic Veterinarians. What is most important is that you find a vet that will listen to and value your concerns in the way you want your pet treated.

I was fortunate enough to work with a veterinarian and university that often thought outside the box when treating pets. Rather than only using traditional and often toxic remedies for the treatment of animals, all options were on the table. I remember one case in particular involving an elderly gentleman and his equally elderly k-9 companion. One afternoon the clinic door opened and after a long pause a very old little black dog slowly entered taking tiny painful steps, followed by an elderly man walking in much the same way. The two had shared many years together and were both feeling the effects of time on their bodies. The elderly gentleman approached the counter and in a sad voice said that he needed to speak to the Vet about letting his friend go as his joints ached, he was incontinent, and his mind was slipping. And his poor little dog was having all the same problems. The old man reluctantly talked to the vet, who was a very compassionate man and knew how hard it would be for the man to lose his companion, so he suggested giving him enough time to contact the local university where he often consulted, to see if they might know of something that could be done instead of putting the little dog to sleep. The university told the vet about a new therapy they were studying using phosphatidylcholine (an essential fatty acid available in any drug store) in elderly animals. They were seeing amazing results, not only with cognitive function but they found it was also helping with arthritis and incontinence. So, the vet gave the elderly gentleman the phosphatidylcholine pills to give to his little dog for a few weeks to see if there would be any improvement. At the very least it might give them a little more time together. Well about three weeks later the clinic door opened and immediately the little black dog came running in, very excited, followed by a long pause until finally the elderly gentleman was able to make his way through the door behind him, every step he took causing him pain. He slowly walked up to the counter and gratefully related how well his little dog was doing. It was like he was young again. The incontinence was gone and he was becoming more and more playful. He said that the only reason he had returned was to find out how he could "get some of whatever that stuff was" for himself! The transformation in the little black dog was amazing. Nearly 20 years later it was reported in the news that phosphatidylcholine was showing great promise in the treatment of Alzheimer's patients.[291] By approaching a vet that respects your concerns and truly cares for your little one, you will open up the possibilities for life-changing treatments and a happy, healthy critter.

Garage

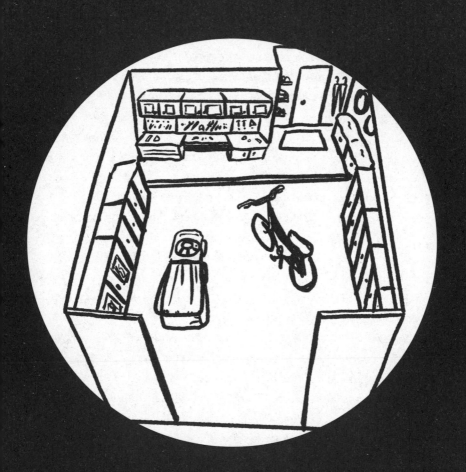

*T*he extra space in the garage is often the place many people use for storage, tools, lawn care items, and on that rare occasion, maybe even as a place to keep their car safe from the elements. Considering this mixture, there are quite a few precautions you can take to reduce toxic risks. For example, if you store gasoline, oil, or other flammable items in your garage you may want to keep them in an insulated storage chest to minimize temperature changes and prevent any fumes from escaping. Another tip is to never run your car in the garage for longer than necessary, as the carbon monoxide exhaust fumes can be brought into your home from the furnace intake fan.

Fire Alarms

As mentioned earlier there are two types of fire alarms. An ionizing fire alarm is designed to respond to a fast flame fire like you might see when storing petroleum products or other flammable chemicals; therefore this would be the best choice for your garage.

Pest Control

It's important to maintain pest control in the garage as it is often more secluded than the rest of the home, and is sometimes used for storing extra food, which can be a magnet for rodents. For every mouse or rat that you see, there are usually many more of them hiding in the corners. There are a couple of humane solutions for eliminating these tenacious little beasts such as live traps, which involve relocation and, to some extent, handling of what is usually a very frightened creature. Then there is the plug-in ultrasonic pest repelling units, which can take up to two weeks to show results and may affect pets living in your home. Then there are many lethal traps. Some are quick and deadly, like the time-honored mouse traps of the late 1800's. The updated version is completely enclosed so that the executioner doesn't even have to see the offending varmint. The one that I have trouble with is the sticky paper, which ensures the long agonizing death of an admittedly very intelligent creature, albeit a pest nonetheless. There is another solution that is humane and effective: rodents, and even insects, hate the smell of peppermint and lemon citrus essential oils. So, by combining food-grade **diatomaceous earth** and the **essential oil** of your choice, you can effectively ward off the little buggers. To do this you will need about a cup of diatomaceous earth and about 1/8 cup of water and either peppermint or lemon citrus essential oil. Add the essential oil (5–7 drops) to the water and mix, then slowly mix in the diatomaceous earth. Place this mixture around the areas you have seen or heard pests and rodents or have found their droppings. It will not harm them, they are repelled by the smell and will leave. The scent will eventually fade from the mixture but can be refreshed by adding a few more drops of oil and a little water. Store any unused mixture in an airtight container for use in the future.

Yard and Garden

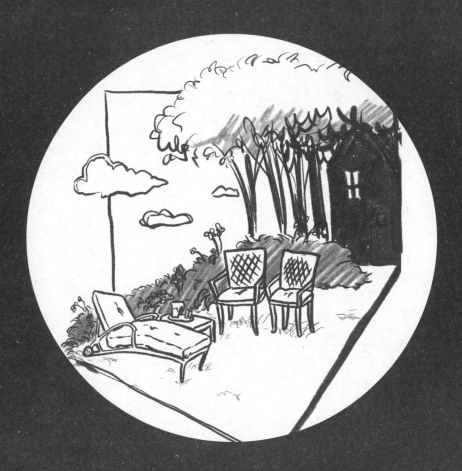

*T*his is an area where, once again, the quest for progress has led to more unforeseen health implications, taking us further away from the earth's natural state. The fresh air, sunshine, and even the soil all have tremendous health benefits. Clean breathing, vitamin D, building allergy resistance, and even the color green has been shown to improve mood and have a calming effect.[292] With many homes having smaller or even tiny yards, you may consider a container garden, and some homes with larger front yards have been opting for nicely landscaped vegetable gardens in front of their house. Whatever your yard provides the following chapter will offer the potential benefits to pursue or toxins to avoid in the process.

Lawn Care

A lawn, or grassy space, absorbs and filters rainwater, provides oxygen, traps dirt, prevents erosion, and provides a cooling effect in the summer. How you grow your lawn can determine whether it is healthy or a health hazard. Lawn pesticides and herbicides make landscaping and growing a garden an easy job, but the problem is that they do not break down as we had been told, and are linked with birth defects, reproductive effects, neurotoxicity, liver or kidney damage, disruption of the endocrine (hormonal) system, and cancer.[293] Children are even more vulnerable than adults as they weigh less, are still developing, and are less able to detoxify. These chemicals can increase a child's likelihood of developing asthma, and have been linked to hyperactivity, developmental delays, behavioral disorders, and motor dysfunction.[294] You can have a nice healthy lawn without the use of all those chemicals. A few tips are:

- Make sure to plant the recommended grass variety for your specific area, taking into account the amount of sun and shade in your yard.

- Do not mow it shorter than two and a half inches during the summer, to prevent the soil from drying out. At the end of the growing season, cut a little shorter to prevent mold from developing over the winter.

- Water about one inch a week, ideally in the early morning.

- Compost it with grass clippings, it provides fertilizer and helps to lighten the soil.

- Keep it small, it is easier to care for, still provides pleasing landscaping and will allow you to use leftover space for a garden. Another advantage to a small lawn is the ability to use a push mower to cut it, which are relatively quiet, non-polluting, and leave the grass greener than a power mower because they shear the grass instead of tearing it.

Organic Gardening

There are many reasons to plant an organic garden. Besides producing healthy food for you and your family, organic gardens are good for the environment. It will save you money on the produce you would normally have to purchase, and your vegetables will be picked fresh so they will retain more nutrients and flavor than store bought. Children benefit greatly from gardening: they not only learn many valuable lessons about nature and how it works, but they develop an appreciation and desire for real food that doesn't come in a box. Even if you have very limited space there are things you can do. Vegetables can be planted in vertical planters, hanging baskets, portable pots, and you can even grow strawberries in a rain gutter (though not while it is attached to the roof). Converting your front and back yards into edible landscaping, using organic and no-till soil regenerative gardening methods, is another way to use the space you have. Organic and no-till gardening methods save water, dramatically reduce weeds, and promote a natural soil population of earthworms and beneficial microbes to ensure a healthy garden. Tilling disrupts and destroys soil biology, but by adding crop cover like mulch or wood chips, it acts as insulation, prevents soil erosion, and also allows soil microbes to thrive. Include pollinator friendly plants in your organic garden. This is important for the success of your crops and good for the bees. If you purchase plants for this purpose make sure they have not been pretreated with pesticides that are toxic to bees, as some sold in nurseries contain neonicotinoids.[295]

Raised Bed Gardens

If you make a raised bed garden, it is best not to use cinder blocks in the construction, as these blocks are made using fly ash, which contains high levels of heavy metals including arsenic, lead, mercury, cadmium, chromium and selenium, as well as aluminum, antimony, barium, beryllium, boron, chlorine, cobalt, manganese, molybdenum, nickel, thallium, vanadium, and zinc.[296] These poisons can leach into the soil and any plants in the garden. It is also important to avoid using railroad ties, since these are treated with arsenic and creosote,[297] a chemical shown to cause cancer.[298] Even touching creosote is considered dangerous. If you do your research on the subject of railroad ties, you might find conflicting information. Some sources say that if the ties are old enough much of the toxins will have already deteriorated and you may find many chain stores selling them for the purpose of landscaping and garden use. These chain stores usually carry a warning label as to the possible carcinogenic chemicals used on the ties but normally you will only see it on their website. Even pressure treated wood contains potentially toxic chemicals. So, if you are using them in landscaping where children might be playing on them, or in a garden where the chemicals might seep into the plants you are growing, you may want to be on the safe side and avoid them all together.

Natural rocks or untreated wood such as cedar, redwood, or cypress are all better options.

Garden Hose

You work very hard to make sure that your lawn and garden are safe and nontoxic for your family. However, that garden hose you are using to water it may sabotage your efforts. Most hoses are made from polyvinyl chloride, phthalates, BPA, bromine, antimony, lead, and organotins. Besides the actual hose itself, the metal fixtures and connectors can also contain heavy metals as well. When these hoses are in the sun the chemicals leach out and into the water. There are safe garden hoses available, such as natural rubber hoses, which are good for gardening but not rated drinking water safe. The best are garden hoses labeled "drinking water safe," "lead free," and "BPA-free." Be sure to store your hose in a cool dark place, as sunlight can break down the hose regardless of what it is made from.

Insecticide

If you find that even with all your natural gardening techniques you still have a few uninvited guests showing up there are a few things you can do. For aphids, mites, whiteflies, and the like:

- A handful of **mint**

- 5-7 cloves of **garlic**

- **Water** as needed

- 1 tbsp **cayenne**

- **Castile soap**

Blend up mint and garlic, adding enough water to liquify.

Pour mixture into a cooking pan, add cayenne pepper, and stir until it comes to a boil.

Remove the mixture from the stove and allow it to cool overnight.

Add a squirt of castile soap and stir.

Pour through a strainer into a spray bottle and spray on affected plants as needed. I have found it to be very effective.

Alternatively, you can mix one cup of **vegetable oil** with one tablespoon of **castile soap** and store. To use, add two teaspoons of this mixture to one quart of **water** in a spray bottle. Shake before spraying plants as needed. Take care to rinse your plants thoroughly prior to eating them. **Diatomaceous earth** is another great nontoxic pesticide. Basically fossilized algae, diatomaceous earth doesn't poison bugs but rather dehydrates them to death. Sprinkle it around your garden to control snails and slugs. Even ants and fleas are repelled by this natural substance.

On the other hand, not all bugs are bad, in fact some are even beneficial for your garden. Ladybugs, easily purchased at most garden stores, will eat mites and aphids. Praying mantises and lacewings are also very effective pest deterrents. Nematodes are another beneficial insect available in garden centers: the microscopic eggs are mixed with water and added to the soil to protect against cutworms, beetles, fleas, and root weevil larvae.

Weed Killer/Herbicide

Glyphosate is found in every corner of the world, and while there are studies to suggest that glyphosate is safe, there are just as many to suggest that it is not. In fact, in 2015 the World Health Organization's International Agency for Research on Cancer (IARC) declared that glyphosate is "probably carcinogenic."[299]

For a **natural herbicide alternative**, mix one half gallon of white vinegar with one half cup of salt then add a squirt of dish soap (castile soap is best). Shake it up until the salt is dissolved and pour it into a spray bottle. I have used this to get rid of weeds that grow in the cracks and crevasses of the driveway and it is very effective. However, unlike glyphosate, it may require additional spraying when new weeds start to grow.

Fertilizer

One popular source of organic fertilizer is herbivore manure. Horses, cows, rabbits, and chicken manure are among the best. Our free-range chickens eat earwigs and other bugs that would otherwise eat our garden, as well as leaving fertilizer behind in the process. If there are any horse stables around, you will usually find that the owner will be more than happy to let you "muck out a stable" and take the resulting "fertilizer" home for free. While great for any garden, horse fertilizer is particularly amazing for your roses. Compost is another great source of fertilizer. There is no expense involved and it is recycling at its best. When you add compost to the soil it adds beneficial microorganisms that increase earthworm activity in your soil. Worm castings (or manure) provide nutrients to the soil and even more beneficial microorganisms that break down organic matter into a form that plant roots can intake. There's also seaweed, which is not only good for the soil but also acts as a natural slug repellent. The same is true of coffee grounds, though they are usually already in the compost. Epsom salt may seem an unlikely fertilizer however it is very helpful when growing tomatoes and peppers. Epsom salt is not really a salt but a magnesium rich mineral compound that helps the plants to grow larger, tastier produce. Just mix a tablespoon with a gallon of water and spray or pour around the base of the plant. You can even mix the Epsom salt crystals directly into the soil if desired, they will dissolve as the plant is watered.

Attics and Basements

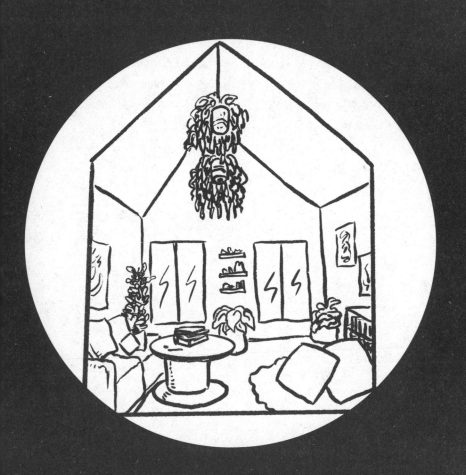

Oftentimes these rooms are finished with particle board, which can off-gas dangerous chemicals such as formaldehyde. While most people do not spend a lot of time in either of these places, the air from these rooms can be circulated throughout the house by heating or air conditioning vents. Therefore, it is important to make sure these areas are free of mold or chemicals you want to avoid.

Insulation

Essential to keeping your home warm in the winter or cool in the summer, there are several kinds of insulation:

Fiberglass: the most commonly used in homes in the US. It can cause skin or eye irritation on contact, and if it is inhaled can cause coughing, nose bleeds, and other respiratory issues. Not to mention, if fiberglass insulation is not properly sealed, it can release tiny fibers into the air.[300] *Cellulose:* usually made from recycled newspaper, it is chemically treated to prevent insects, fungi, bacteria, and combustion.

Spray polyurethane foam: insulates better than fiberglass or cellulose and is energy efficient. This type of insulation contains chemical fumes that are dangerous until the foam has fully expanded and dried completely.[301]

The Alternatives: Sheep's **wool insulation** is one of the most natural and renewable resources available, and it comes with many benefits.[302] It does not require any special protective equipment for installation, and is naturally fire resistant. While other forms of insulation tend to settle over time, wool instead expands and can even absorb dangerous chemicals that may be in your walls.[303] The best part is that it is very effective, as proven by its R-value, the rating used by the department of energy to measure resistance to the flow of heat through a given thickness of a material (such as insulation). For example, cellulose has an average rating of R3.5, foam insulation is about R5, and wool *starts* at R4 while many of the brands available on the internet are R13–R19, depending on cost.

Radon Danger

Radon is a cancer-causing, naturally occurring radioactive gas produced by decaying uranium. You cannot see, smell, or taste radon, but it may be a problem in your home, as elevated radon levels have been found in every state in the US.[304] Radon in the soil, groundwater, or building materials enters working and living spaces. It can seep directly through pores in the concrete, but also from gaps in the walls or floors, especially in the basement. Elevated levels of radon can be found in any house in any state. There are several testing options for your home. Short term tests are available at most home improvement stores. They are simple to use, simply measure detectable Radon by setting the test out for two to seven days and then mail the test to a lab for results. According to the EPA if the test registers 4 picoCuries per liter or higher of Radon then a second test should be done. A long term test will measure Radon levels for three months to one year. As many factors can affect these levels such as air pressure, wind, soil moisture, and even snow cover, which may trap the gases, this is considered a more accurate testing method. There are also continuous testing monitors that provide a running average by continually sampling the air using an ionizing chamber. Reducing radon levels in your home can be done in a variety of ways, some as simple as increasing ventilation or sealing cracks in floors and walls. However if this is not sufficient you should call a qualified contractor with the specific skills and knowledge to correct the problem.

Mold

Mold is most prevalent in basements or attics. Sometimes it can be identified by a musty odor or you may even see black splotches covering areas of the walls or ceiling. The spores produced by the mold can become airborne and cause a myriad of health issues.[305] If you find a small area that is affected, it can be cleared up using hydrogen peroxide and baking soda to remove the offending stain. Another alternative that can be found in any home improvement store is Concrobium. It is available in a spray bottle or in gallon jugs to be used in a fogging machine for room size areas. According to the MSDS (material data safety sheet) this product is not considered hazardous and is very effective at removing mold.[306] If however a large area is affected, for example from flood damage or constant damp conditions, an expert should be consulted. If you are not sure if mold is an issue there are test kits available from most home improvement stores.

Shopping for Alternatives

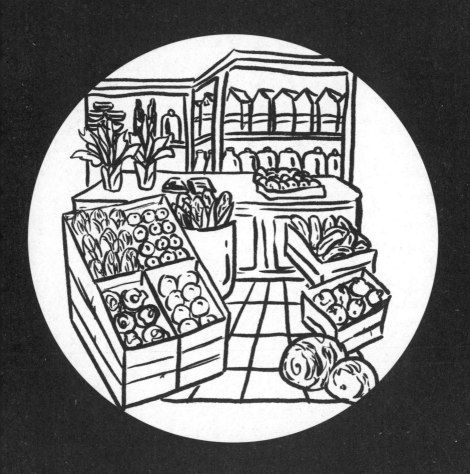

*T*he internet is full of useful and not so useful information. When researching on any subject it is important to check the source of the information to see if they have a dog in the fight, so to speak. Some corporations even pay individuals to write bogus blogs or misleading articles about subjects to influence the reader toward their monetary gain. For example: if you research articles about cannabis you may notice a negative bias from websites connected to the pharmaceutical industry and positive articles from the more natural healing websites. That is why you will want to check several websites on a subject and check the sources. When shopping for products it is important to remember that just because something is labeled "natural," "eco-friendly," or "green," it doesn't mean it is nontoxic. The regulations and guidelines that determine the definition of these terms change depending on the success of the lawyers and lobbyists responsible for molding these definitions . This is also true in connection to food; organic and non-GMO standards are changing constantly. In fact, something can be labeled as non-GMO even if it is not since the FDA states that refined products that come from GMO sources, such as oil made from soy or canola will not have to be labeled as containing GMO ingredients. You have to learn to read between the lines and all of the fine print. If something says grass fed but not 100% grass fed, then it most likely means that it was grain finished (fed grain for the last few months of its life) and could be GMO grain finished.

Ingredients

When you are making your own products, it is important to remember that what you end up with will only be as good as the ingredients you used to make it. The source of your ingredients can make all the difference in the world as to how effective your products end up being. An example of this is cinnamon. Ceylon cinnamon is believed to help treat type 2 diabetes, lower bad cholesterol, help with Alzheimer's symptoms, and fight inflammation. However, the most commonly used form of cinnamon is Cassia cinnamon, as it is the least expensive and the easiest to obtain. The problem here is that Cassia cinnamon does not contain the same health benefits as Ceylon cinnamon, according to research. So those who are using the standard form of available cinnamon in grocery stores for health benefits but not seeing any results think that it must just not work, when in reality they are simply using the wrong source for their purpose.[307] Of course, when shopping for ingredients, choosing organic over conventional is always a better choice for those wanting to avoid toxic pesticides and glyphosate.

Essential oil: Essential oils can greatly enhance your personal care and cleaning products. The source of the oils you use is critical, and this is where labels are *very* important. Some things you should look for are the Latin name of the plant used. There are many different types of each plant, like the cinnamon example seen above, so make sure it is the correct source. It should state the country of origin, as this is also important in determining the quality. It should also indicate the purity. An example comes to mind of a bottle of myrrh with a label that read 100% pure and natural, then at the bottom in small print said 20% oil blend. It should say 100% pure essential oil of myrrh. Remember that, while good quality essential oils are not cheap, they are very effective, potent, will go a long way, and last a long time.

Note: Remember that essential oils are very potent and should always be diluted with a carrier oil when used on the skin. Citrus essential oils such as grapefruit, orange, and lemon may increase your photosensitivity and should be avoided before sun exposure. Many essential oils are toxic to pets.

Activated charcoal: This product has many uses both internally and externally. It can be used for whitening teeth, added to facial masks, as a wound dressing, or even to treat bug bites. It can be purchased in bulk or in capsule form, and, as with any product, it is important to consider the source. Charcoal comes from many places. The most absorbent, which is what you want, comes from organic raw materials, like organically grown coconut or wood. Avoid the ones that do not list the materials used in making the product or any that contain additives. Activated charcoal will not stain your skin but can be challenging to remove from clothing, so use caution when you are mixing it or using it on your skin. If it does get on your clothes just pre-soak the area with a little castile soap before washing and you should be fine.

Conclusion

Does One Cup Make a Difference?

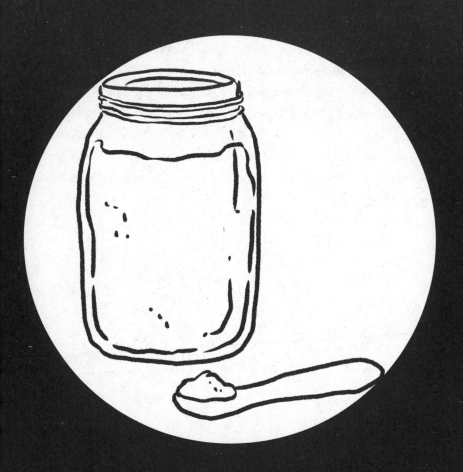

From the moment we get up in the morning our choices have an impact. The things you do have an effect on the world around you. The purchases you make support companies whose policies help shape the world now, and to come. Something as small as your morning cup of coffee can have a significant impact. Is it organic, fair trade, and shade grown? Does it matter?

Well, choosing organic coffee means that you will not be drinking the residue of synthetic chemicals, fertilizers, fungicides, herbicides, and pesticides that are sprayed on every acre of non-organic coffee.[308] Not to mention that non-organic coffee is grown by farmers that are exposed to high levels of toxic chemicals. They are not the only ones affected, as the surrounding communities are also impacted by the residue of all of these toxins as they end up in the air and water.[309]

Large coffee growers also cut down huge swaths of rainforest in order to have more room to increase production (the same rain forest that produces over 20% of the world's oxygen).[310] This deforestation destroys the natural habitat of the local wildlife that maintains balance within the ecosystem. Without these natural pest deterrents, the coffee-loving bugs take over, leading to the use of more and more pesticides. Then when it rains, the lack of trees leads to soil erosion, and the resulting water runoff carries the toxic chemicals into the water supply of the surrounding areas. Instead, shade grown means the coffee beans were grown in a forested area, with all the natural pest controlling animals that produce natural fertilizer, making it safer for the farmer, community, and you.

Many of the changes you make can have a huge impact, and yet require very little effort. I purchase organic, fair trade, shade grown coffee from Trader Joes or Costco for the same price as most conventionally grown coffee.

You can usually find it at any natural food store or even order it online. I add organic grass-fed half-and-half and organic sugar or stevia and drink it in a ceramic mug. This way, I haven't contributed to the demise of the environment or farmers, I haven't supported factory farms or GMO crops, and I haven't added to the plastic in the oceans. Most coffee shops offer organic options so even if you get your cup of joe on the way to work, you can keep your commitment to a healthier planet, especially if you bring your own container.

This is just one example to show you how the little changes you make in your home and lifestyle can keep you and your family free of some of the worst toxins we're surrounded by on a daily basis. When you buy organic fair trade products, you are not only making sure that the farmer is receiving a living wage for his labor, but helping to ensure environmental sustainability, since most fair-trade farmers use production methods that will keep the natural environment thriving for generations to come.

So yes, I would say that one cup of coffee does make a difference.

AFTERWORD
Tried and True Nontoxic Products

In this day and age, it seems everyone is incredibly busy, and while I have endeavored to include recipes for alternatives to most of the toxic products listed in this book, I am aware that most individuals do not have the time to create the products mentioned throughout. So, I did my best to research companies dedicated to providing products that were safe for those using them as well as having a commitment to animal welfare and the environment. I'm sharing what I have found to be the best brands and places to purchase them, but that of course does not mean you might not do better yourself. It should be noted that I receive no compensation for any of the products that I share in this book and I have included them purely because I use them myself and trust the company that is selling them.

On that note, it is important to remember that companies occasionally sell out to big corporations that will keep the name of the brand but may change the ingredients. For example, Tom's of Maine, known for using only natural ingredients, was bought out by Colgate. It can be a challenge to keep up with, but it is well worth the effort.

I started my research with the Environmental Working Group website: they test and rate everything from baby formula, water, and personal care products, to pet foods. If you have a question about a product, their website is a good place to start. They even have an app for that: EWG's Healthy Living App. You just scan the barcode of a product and they rate allergy, cancer, and developmental concerns, then list all of the ingredients and give a summary of the findings. As more people become aware of the health and environmental implications of their choices, companies are taking notice. The result is more widely available choices for consumers.

The following list is only a starting point, as Natural and Health food stores, and careful internet research are good sources for supplies or ready to use products.

Home & Personal Care

100% Pure: providing cosmetics colored with plant pigments. It is one of the very few cosmetic companies I have found to not use heavy metals or artificial colors in the line. After doing extensive research I currently use this company as my source for lipstick and mascara. Their commitment to providing a healthy, high quality product is evident in the ingredients they use and processing methods they employ. The products are available in some retail locations as seen on the website, or can be ordered online at 100percentpure.com

Akar: a very high-quality skin regimen inspired by Tibet's natural beauty. They source traditional ingredients such as sea buckthorn and goji berries from Tibet, as well as organic and wildcrafted ingredients from growers who care for our earth. The products detoxify, balance, and restore your skin's natural beauty. With a vision to provide their customers with beautiful, effective skincare, that happens to be 100% natural and free from toxins. All of the products including the Lip Butter are housed in dark glass containers, which protects the ingredients inside from breaking down in sunlight and prevents leaching from plastic. Using the products makes you feel like you have been to a spa. You might think that adding oils to your face would cause excessive shine or blemishes, but the opposite is true with akar: my skin felt soft and nourished. It takes a very small amount of the oil to accomplish a well-balanced healthy glowing complexion. The Lip Butter was very hydrating and lasted for hours. Akar is EWG verified, environmentally conscious, and animal friendly. Worldwide shipping is available from their website akarskin.com

Arganat: a company that goes beyond just offering nontoxic personal care products. Made for all genders and skin types, their products incorporate the renewal of ancient knowledge from African, European, and native cultures of the world, and are made in Montréal. The founder created this line of products, supported by her background as a biochemist, environmentalist, and naturopath, to offer powerful, harmless products able to rejuvenate skin. The core ingredients of Arganat are organic extra virgin argan oil and ultra ventilated clays (ARGile (clay) +ARGan oil +NATurel =Arganat) with wild and organic essential oils, medicinal plants, and virgin cold pressed vegetable oils, making all the products edible. They are chemical free, eco-friendly, and do not test on animals, and mostly vegan. Unlike the most common drawback to the "all natural" products, they smell wonderful. They seem to surpass even the high end (toxic) facial care lines available in retail stores with safe, listed ingredients that are much less expensive while being effective beyond their promises. I used their toothpaste and several of the facial treatments for two weeks and was impressed by them all. The toothpaste was clay based, had a pleasant taste, and a list of very healing ingredients. It has a gentle whitening effect as well as improving gum health. The Facial Tonifying Cleanser also contains a small amount of clay, combined with argan oil and a few other ingredients, which cleans and tones in one step. Followed up with the Fountain of Youth Serum to brighten, tone, and reduce fine lines, it leaves your skin feeling soft and smooth. The Power Cream is great for any areas of dry skin; it will leave your hands silky smooth, and I found it to be an excellent lip gloss. Arganat is EWG verified, dedicated to protecting the environment, and animal friendly. The products are available worldwide from the website arganat.net

Be Green Bath & Body: artisanal, natural and organic skin care. This company provides affordable nontoxic products for the whole family from head to toe. Including skin care for every skin type, shower gels, deodorants, shaving foam, a variety of creams, and every baby care product you could possibly need. Be Green has an extensive line of available products that will allow you to replace almost every toxic personal care product in your bathroom. They have a very nice deodorant bar, lightly scented, suitable for adults and children, and it takes only a little to be effective all day. The Calendula cream is said to be good for relieving eczema, but I have a friend who successfully used it on a sore foot to relieve pain. I use the miracle balm in place of Neosporin, and the shaving foam is light and silky, always leaving my legs free of nicks. While I have tried many of their products and found them all to be of good quality and effective, I have to say my favorite is their rosehip Regenerative Serum. This serum contains frankincense and helichrysum oils, among other ingredients, to create a wonderfully hydrating, healing oil. This family-owned business has been making nontoxic personal care products since 2008. All of their products are made in small batches to ensure freshness. They are highly rated by EWG, cruelty free, they support the Savvy Women's Alliance, and have earned Green America's Green Business Certification. Their products are available from their website at begreenbathandbody.com

Bite: an all natural, plastic free way to replace your toothpaste. In an effort to reduce the one billion (with a B) toothpaste tubes thrown away every year and provide a healthy alternative to the chemicals used in conventional toothpaste, Bite is committed to providing a brighter smile that doesn't come at the expense of our bodies or the environment. They use clean cruelty free ingredients to create tablets, inventing a whole new convenient, no-waste way to achieve oral hygiene. All you do is place a Bite tablet in your mouth and bite down then brush with a wet toothbrush, the tablet foams up releasing the ingredients that, along with the brushing action, cleans your teeth and freshens your breath. The small tablets are supplied in a small glass reusable/ recyclable bottle and shipped using recycled paper products. I have used these myself as well as sharing them with others and found them to be refreshing, effective, and fun to use. Everyone who tried them agreed and added that they are very convenient and would be great for traveling. Available online at bitetoothpastebits.com

Boyzz Only: made with high quality natural and organic ingredients. As the name implies this is a product line marketed towards men and boys. It includes shampoo, conditioner, detangler, and hair and body wash in scented or unscented varieties. The products are EWG verified and bear the Certclean logo, which means they are free from ingredients that may pose a risk to hormonal, reproductive, or neurological systems. Boyzz Only is created by QNaturals, a small family owned company in the foothills of the Canadian Rockies. All of the products are vegan, cruelty free, and environmentally friendly and the packaging looks amazing. I had the hair and body wash tested by a few people and they all came back with rave reviews. While it is a product of Canada and available in some retail stores as seen on the website, it is available online for the rest of us. Check them out online at boyzzonly.com.

Chagrin Valley Soap & Salve: a small family owned and operated company dedicated to crafting high quality, healthy, and effective skin and hair care products that will nourish your skin and be kind to our planet. Their ingredients are certified organic, sustainably produced, cruelty-free, and ethically traded. They carry a large variety of products for adults, children, and even pets. I have only tried a few of their products. The Bug-Off stick, which I can highly recommend, is easy to carry, easy to use, and best of all it works to keep the bugs at bay. The Goldenseal Myrrh Herbal Salve is a great nontoxic alternative for antibiotic ointment used for cuts and scrapes. And the Mint Mist Coconut Cream Deodorant, with a bamboo spatula applicator, takes very little to do the job and has a wonderful light scent. They also have deodorants in stick form. The products are affordable, vegan, cruelty free, and environmentally friendly. Even their packaging is 99% plastic free. Enjoy their website at chagrinvalleysoapandsalve.com

Definitive Rose: providing high end natural skin care products for everyone. All of their products are hand blended, one batch at a time, using herbs and flowers that are organically grown or wildcrafted. All of the products are created under the supervision of a certified master Herbalist to ensure they will deliver verifiable results. I tried these products for myself: the facial cleaner, toner, serum, polish, mask, cream, and eye cream. I was very impressed with the quality and results. After only using them for one week there was a noticeable difference in my skin, especially around my eyes where the skin was tighter, more even toned and, unless it was my hopeful imagination, there were fewer fine lines. Everything about this company is impressive, from the glass containers most of the products come in to the quality of the contents. Definitive Rose has created nontoxic versions of the high-end skin care lines typically found in designer department and clothing stores, and done so at an affordable cost to the consumer. All of the ingredients are listed on their website, they are EWG verified, cruelty free, and dedicated to giving back to the community. While their products are not available in retail stores, they can be ordered from the website definitiverose.com

Derma E: with a passion for health, wellness, and environmental sustainability using vegan, cruelty free formulas since 1984. They provide a variety of skin and body care products free of parabens, SLS, petroleum, mineral oil, or artificial colors, and treat a wide range of conditions from Therapeutic Topicals to the Anti-Wrinkle Collection. I have tried two of their products: the Tea Tree and Vitamin E Antiseptic Cream and the Anti-Wrinkle Cream. Both are quickly absorbed, leaving your skin silky smooth. The products are available at many retail locations including Whole Foods and Walgreens, as well as others that can be seen on their website at dermae.com

Dr. Bronners: providing nontoxic products for nearly every household and personal care purpose, using fair trade, organic, vegan and cruelty free ingredients, and promoting environmental sustainability. Most of their products are available at retail stores everywhere but if you are unable to locate a product needed it can be ordered from their website at drbronner.com

The Essential Oil Company: my hands down favorite place to purchase essential oils. The owner and founder, Robert Seidel, started the company more than 40 years ago and his commitment to producing the highest quality products is unsurpassed. He oversees every aspect of the production process, from growing the raw materials and distillation methods, to ensuring the equipment is properly maintained. But his commitment doesn't stop there. He sources his oils from all over the world, first by traveling to the region where the ingredients are grown and harvested to meet with the local people that will be providing the oils. He works to provide many local makers with a sustainable livelihood that also has a positive impact on the environment. Because the oils are globally sourced, some are certified organic, some are organic but not certified, and some are wildcrafted in areas that are free of pesticides and herbicides. The resulting oils are used by herbalists, naturopaths, chiropractors, medical doctors, and are available to the public. The Essential Oil Company is based in Portland, Oregon, and can be purchased directly from their headquarters or ordered for worldwide delivery from their informative website at essentialoil.com

Finally Pure: dedicated to making pure, natural, nutrient-rich, organic, and safe products affordable and available to everyone. Every ingredient found in their products is 100% natural and has a high safety rating on the toxin/hazard scale of the Skin Deep Database (part of the EWG website). Because Finally Pure is so safe, it is even being sold in some Medical Centers and being used by people who have, or are recovering from cancer. The products they offer include pregnancy and baby lotions, oils, soaps, and lip balms for children and adults. As children often ingest most lip balms, it is a comfort to be confident of its safety. I tried the Jelly Bean Lip Balm which smelled just like Jelly Beans and was very smooth and moisturizing when applied. It would be a very nice solution for your little ones' chapped lips on a cold day. They also make body lotions, soap, and washes as well as everything for the face. I have tried two of the body lotions, and they are soothing and moisturizing. One is the Rosemary mint hand and body lotion, the other, Finally for Pregnancy hand and body lotion. I let my pregnant friend try this one to relieve itchy skin on her ever-expanding stomach, and it worked like a charm. Finally Pure is EWG verified, cruelty free, and Green Business Certified. You can order from their website at finallypure.com

Force of Nature: a nontoxic cleaner as effective as bleach with no toxic chemicals. It comes as a kit, with an activator base, an activator bottle, five capsules containing salt, water, and vinegar, a 12-ounce spray bottle and a 2-ounce spray bottle. When you follow the simple directions you will have a powerful nontoxic cleaner and disinfectant within minutes. The kit can be ordered online with free shipping at forceofnatureclean.com

Homestead Body: a company founded by a husband and wife team on the principle of going back to the basics for clean body care. Committed to using the finest organic fair trade certified ingredients, their products are unisex, certified vegan, and cruelty free. A portion of each sale is donated to animal rescue. The products are reasonably priced and include face and body oils and butters, rub deodorants, clay masks, exfoliants, soaking salts, and even beard oils. I have used the Butterlove Body Butter and found the fluffy texture absorbed quickly and kept my skin hydrated for hours. They make a very effective baking soda free deodorant rub for those who are sensitive. The Skin Love Body Oil is a wonderful all over moisturizer and great for use after dry brushing your skin, and they also sell it as a kit with the oil and brush. They offer free samples on request from their website at homesteadbody.com

Just the Goods: a website focused on healthier, handmade alternatives to mass produced chemicals, using vegetable and mineral based ingredients with known track records. It's about accessibility and affordability. On the website you will find a complete line of handmade personal care products for adults and children. They also carry cosmetics by The All Natural Face, aromatherapeutic candles by Mother Earth Essentials, and nail polish by Suncoat, to name just a few. There are sample sizes available, great for travel or curiosity about a product, which is how I tried the "about face" skin care kit. It left my skin clean without drying it out, the moisturizer absorbed quickly without any greasy feeling, and the kit included lip balm with a nice peppermint scent. I also tried some of the hair products: the leave in spray conditioner and deep conditioning treatment. Both gave very nice results to hydrate my otherwise dry hair. The anti-frizz serum was incredibly effective; it takes very little to add shine and tame the frizz. The shaving solids contain avocado oil which is great for reducing age spots and sun damage.[311] They make a vegan perfume available in several fragrances. I sampled wild woods scent and even added it to the anti-frizz serum which made my hair smell nice as well. They also carry gift sets with meditation gemstones, incense, and matcha tea. Just the Goods is EWG verified, vegan, cruelty free, and environmentally friendly. The website for products available worldwide is justthegoods.net

Lowen's: a family owned business based in Canada, led by a veteran Pharmacist committed to using organic, fair-trade, and locally-sourced ingredients to produce skin care products that are safe, effective, and affordable. Lowen's Natural Skincare is inspired by, and named after their daughter, Lowen. After unsuccessful attempts to treat their daughter's diaper rash using commercially available products they decided to develop their own natural diaper balm using proven, safe ingredients. The resulting formula permanently resolved their baby's diaper rash. Hoping to help others in the same situation they started Lowen's, which now creates a variety of balms, lotions, cleaners, scrubs, and creams. All of their products are thoroughly evaluated for safety, effectiveness, environmental impact, and animal welfare by the EWG and PETA. They have created a product called Vegan Vaporub which is the best replacement for its toxic counterpart I have found yet. It was comforting to know that when my son was rubbing it all over his chest he wasn't adding dangerous chemicals to his skin while trying to recover from a cold. It allowed him to breathe easier and cough less, getting a good night's sleep without the toxic, greasy, petroleum ingredients. They also make very moisturizing lip balms in a large variety of flavors suitable for all ages. I wanted to try the Bum Balm Blues, but as diaper rash is not a problem for me, I used it on my elbows where the skin tends to be dry and can crack. Problem solved by the second day: no more dry skin. I have tried Lowen's Conditioning Shampoo, facial cleaner, and Bubble Bath and have been impressed by each. The Bubble Bath is great for adults but is a must for those with small children who like to play in the tub, since they will not have to worry if any gets in their mouths while splashing around. They make a lotion called Rub it in Why Don't Ya!, which I have shared with others suffering from chapped skin and is loved by all. Lowen's carries many other personal care products as well and is committed to developing more in the future but for now you will find an assortment for adults and children for everything from chapped lips to aiding in the healing of new tattoos. Lowen's products are available in many retail stores in Canada (which are listed in the website provided) but can be ordered directly from their website if you live elsewhere. Delivery is fast and free on orders over $50.00. Their website is lowens.ca

Qet (keet): fresh and effective premium care for face, body, and hair without the use of toxins, synthetics, harmful chemicals, or preservatives. Handcrafted in small fresh batches to keep the integrity and the effectiveness of the ingredients pure and high performing. When I received delivery of the Hair Care Suite and Getting Started Facial Kit, I was first impressed by the beautifully gift-wrapped packaging. I soon learned that the contents were equally impressive. The Hair Care Suite was a godsend for my hair as it is long, curly, and can be difficult to control. The Natural Sea Spray was the first nontoxic curl enhancer

I have ever found. It wasn't heavy or sticky; in fact, except for defrizzing and defining my curls, it felt like there was nothing added to my hair. It was even more effective when used in combination with the Natural Shine Serum and Nuti-Pomade. Curly hair tends to be very dry and frizzy, but these products added shine and control without the harmful ingredients. The Facial Suite Kit products are packaged in small glass containers and come in a zippered carrying case which would be perfect for traveling. They provided me with almost two weeks of cleansing, toning, exfoliating, and moisturizing. I loved the way my skin felt and looked. All of the treatments are EWG verified, and they are a Certified Green Business with Green America. The Qet line is available in some retail stores as shown on their website but can be ordered worldwide from qetbotanicals.com

Sally B's: a company started by the founder who, after recovering from cancer, became dedicated to providing safe personal care products for others. Enlisting the help of a chemist and nutritionist, then spending countless hours on ingredient and cosmetic research, Sally created products without the chemicals and toxins. She provides a wide range of products such as face and body care, make-up, and even deodorant pads. I was very impressed with her Healing Hand Butter as it absorbed quickly and left my hands very soft with no greasy residue. It is a good choice for chapped and tired hands. I also tried the B Glossy Lip Gloss and Lip Skinnies, both were very moisturizing, adding a little color without overpowering and they lasted. The Tamanu Luxury Facial Cleaner removed dirt and makeup without drying out my skin, and the list of mostly organic ingredients allowed me to feel good about what I was putting on my body. Sally B's products are EWG verified, certified cruelty free, and contain the highest concentration of certified organic ingredients possible. They are available in some retail stores throughout the US, as shown on their website, but are also available worldwide at sallybskinyummies.com

Soap for Goodness Sake: a husband and wife team offering handmade soap and body products. The handmade soaps are made with organic base oils, not commercial grade, which can contain other additives. In addition, they use hot springs thermal water and other pure and natural ingredients. I have used three different varieties of the soaps and found all three to be of exceptional quality. They also offer Miessence certified organic products on their website, so you can find anything from makeup, toothpaste, to skin care and hair care products. They are from Australia and have an impressive list of organic ingredients. I have used several. The Desert Flower shampoo is very moisturizing, and they have a mint toothpaste with a nice flavor and whitening effect. They also offer a line of nontoxic nail polish, one of the few I have seen. They are an eco-friendly company and use only sustainable organic plantation palm oil which does not contribute to palm forest destruction. They use 100% PCW chlorine free paper for printing whenever possible as well as eco-friendly packaging. All of the products are available from the website at soapforgoodnesssake.com

Sustain: a company dedicated to providing safe feminine hygiene products. They don't stop there; they also offer nitrosamine-free condoms, organic lubricant, and wipes. The lubricant is pH balanced, vegan, and free of petroleum and other toxic chemicals, safe for pregnancy, toys, and latex. Best of all, it is effective. The tampons are 100% organic cotton, with a plant based (recyclable) applicator. Great performance aside, you can rest assured that you are not absorbing toxic dyes, fragrances, pesticides, or other chemicals in the most sensitive areas of your body. The pads and liners are also 100% organic cotton, they stay put, and provide leak-proof protection. The Ultra-Thin Condoms come in a variety of fits and quantities, and are electronically tested for safety. I was impressed with the quality of the products and the commitment to not only the health of the one using them, but also the health of the environmental impact by the use of the 100% post-consumer recycled paper packaging. The company sources fair trade organic cotton and latex. They also give 10% of their profits to women's healthcare organizations. They are vegan-certified, and, of course, cruelty free. The products are available online at sustainnatural.com

Whole Body Apothecary: a company working to set higher standards in transparency, nutrition and sustainability for the skin care and supplement industries. A fascinating company that provides a variety of products from handmade soaps and salves, deodorants, beard oils, and shaving products to specialized teas and tinctures. When shopping from their website you can shop by category under topics like, Energy & Focus, Anxiety & Sleep, Immune & Recovery, or Dry Skin. I have tried a few of their products, including the lemongrass soap, which has a wonderful fragrance and is not drying. Two deodorants, Lavender and Citrusness, were both very effective, even for highly active individuals. I was impressed with the smooth consistency, as most natural deodorants can feel like you are applying sand paper. It is definitely one of my favorites for performance and price. The Little Buddy salve is a nice addition to the diaper bag, but also useful for any dry, itchy, irritated skin on bodies of all ages. It is also very soothing for chapped lips. Whole Body Apothecary carries a nice variety of herbal tea blends; the formulas based on modernized concepts of Ayurveda. Of these I have tried the Inflammation Tea, Sleepy Tea, and Digestion Tea, and all contained a wonderful array of organic ingredients. The Sleepy Tea was very relaxing and, in my case, aided in an uninterrupted night's sleep. Whole Body Apothecary offers free samples of most of their products and back all purchases with a 100% money-back guarantee. They are cruelty free, and very eco-friendly. Their website is worth checking out at wholebodyapothecary.com

Pet Foods

A proper diet results in many benefits for your pets: healthy weight, shiny coat, improved digestion, more energy, healthy teeth, and relief from allergies. A species specific, nutritionally complete, and, ideally, raw diet is the best food source for any pet. However, making it yourself can be very time consuming, not to mention frustrating, so here are some of my suggestions.

Fresh is Best: providing a variety of grain free freeze-dried dog and cat food. All products are 100% free of grains, white potatoes, peas, and tapioca flours. Only fresh whole fruits and veggies—no dried pomace. No added hormones or antibiotics, all grass-fed beef. Fresh is Best was started when founder Stacy LaPoints' dog, a German Shepherd named Jade, became ill with Addison's disease. Researching pet nutrition and enlisting the help of an animal nutrition scientist, she developed a dog and cat food line able to ensure that the accepted nutrition profiles, as determined by the AAFCO, are met or exceeded in each recipe. You'll be happy to know that as a result Jade lived a happy life until the ripe old age of fourteen. I have fed three varieties of Fresh is Best cat food to my cats; the duck, chicken, and turkey options. While they enjoyed all three, their favorite was the chicken. Fresh is Best is available at retail stores shown on the website but can also be ordered from the website at freshisbest.com

Primal Pet Foods: with a goal to nourish pets the way nature intended, was founded by Matt Koss after his dog was diagnosed with early signs of renal failure. Matt took the advice of a holistic veterinarian who recommended switching his dog to a diet based on bones and raw food. This led to the creation of his own species-appropriate pet food for his dog. After seeing the dramatic improvement in his dog, he set out to bring Primal to the market so that other pets could enjoy a happier, healthier, more vibrant life. They provide a variety of foods for both dogs and cats in raw, frozen, and freeze-dried formulas. In addition to the foods, they also provide bone broth, raw goat milk, bones, and treats. I tried the freeze-dried formulas for my dog and two cats. They were a big hit all around. They were easy to feed, just reconstitute the freeze-dried nuggets with warm water, or to supercharge the meal, add raw goat milk, set the bowl down and stand back. Even my feline finicky eater finished every last morsel. The freeze-dried formulas are great for backpacking or traveling with your pet too. Primal Pet Foods are available from many retail stores, the locations are available on their website, and they can also be ordered from chewy.com

Raw Wild: made from 99.4% organic wild elk and venison and 0.6% vitamins and minerals. Raw Wild has made it easy by providing a complete diet free of fillers, animal byproducts, antibiotics, preservatives, growth hormones, and, best of all, GMO's. The source for the meat is Rocky Mountain grass-fed elk and deer, only producing 1,000 pounds of meat annually. The meat is nutrient dense and, as there are no fillers, your pet will not need to eat as much to be satisfied. As Raw Wild is not available in retail stores and can only be ordered online and delivered to your home. I tried the one-time trial of twelve, one pound packages of what appeared to be very lean ground meat which arrived frozen in a reusable styrofoam chest. It was very easy to feed to my pup; I just defrosted one of the packages and placed about ½ of a pound of the meat in my dog's bowl. She absolutely loved it! Raw Wild Dog Food is formulated to meet the nutritional levels established by the AAFCO Dog Food Nutrient Profiles for dogs for all life stages, including growth of large dogs. It can also be fed to cats if choline and taurine are added. After feeding this to my dog I can wholeheartedly recommend it for yours. It can be ordered from the website at rawwild.com

GLOSSARY

AAFCO: The Association of American Feed Control Officials is a regulatory committee of the sale and distribution of animal feeds (including dog and cat foods) and animal drug remedies.

Allopathic: Pertaining to conventional, western medical treatment of disease.

Bentonite Clay: Bentonite clay is one of the commonly found clays in nature and has been shown to act as a detoxifying agent.

Benzene: This colorless, volatile, liquid hydrocarbon is present in petroleum and coal tar.

Borosilicate: Borosilicate glass is a type of glass mainly composed of silica and boron trioxide, making it less susceptible to thermal shock.

Candida: a genus of yeast-like fungi that are a normal component of the flora of the mouth, skin, intestinal tract, and vagina, but can cause a variety of infections when unchecked.

CFL: Compact Fluorescent Light uses electricity to excite mercury vapor within the glass tube which in turn causes the phosphors and argon gas to glow and produce light.

Circadian rhythms: The diurnal rhythms occurring in organisms that primarily respond to the variations of light and darkness in an organism's environment.

Collagen: a class of extracellular proteins particularly found in the skin, bone, cartilage, tendon, and teeth, that forms strong insoluble fibers and works as connective tissue between cells. When denatured by boiling, collagen will break down into gelatin.

DEA (diethanolamine): A "wetting" agent that is primarily used in shampoos and lotions to provide lather. It can also be found in brake fluid, degreasers, and antifreeze. The chemical is classified by the International Agency for Research on Cancer as "possibly carcinogenic to humans."

Diatomaceous earth: A soft, crumbly, porous sedimentary deposit formed from the fossil remains of diatoms, a species of algae. It is used in skin care products, toothpastes, foods, beverages, medicines, rubbers, paints, and water filters.

Dielectric heating: The way in which microwave ovens heat non-conducting materials by a rapidly varying electromagnetic field that causes the water molecules found within to vibrate at rapid speeds.

Fibromyalgia: is a medical condition that causes pain throughout the body. Other symptoms include sleep problems, fatigue, and even emotional distress. The cause is yet unknown.

Formaldehyde: a colorless, toxic, potentially carcinogenic, water-soluble gas, used as a disinfectant and preservative, and in the manufacture of various resins and plastics.

Genotoxic: a toxic agent that damages DNA molecules, causing mutations and tumors.

Glyphosate: Used as a broad-spectrum herbicide and desiccant for grains, glyphosate can be found in most of the major weed killers used today. It has been linked to an array of health concerns.

GOTS: The Global Organic Textile Standard is the world's premier textile processing standard for organic fibers. It is considered the most rigorous organic textile standard because it goes beyond simply verifying that it was organically farmed to include every step in the manufacturing process.

Histamines: This substance plays a major role in many allergic responses, dilating blood vessels, and increasing the permeability of the vessel walls. In humans, histamine is found in almost all tissues of the body.

Lymphatic system: The system responsible for the production of white blood cells in response to inflammation or presence of antigens.

MEA (Monoethanolamine): Also known as Ethanolamine, MEA is an organic chemical compound primarily used in feedstock and in the production of detergents, emulsifiers, polishes, pharmaceuticals, corrosion inhibitors, and chemical intermediates.

Nebulizers: A device for producing a fine spray of liquid.

Nitrates: A salt or ester of nitric acid. They are used as preservatives and color fixatives in cured meats as well as used for other industrial purposes, such as an ingredient in gunpowder, explosives, fertilizers, and glass enamels.

Nitrosamines: These are carcinogenic organic compounds that have shown to correlate with cancers of the stomach, esophagus, nasopharynx, and urinary bladder. They are formed in the stomach by a reaction between nitrites and the amine groups of certain proteins in food, and can also be found in beer, certain drugs, and cigarette smoke.

PentaBDE: These are brominated hydrocarbons used as flame retardants in everything from plastics to furniture, upholstery, electrical equipment, textiles, and a slew of other household products.

PicoCuries: A measurement used to determine the radioactivity produced by radon gas as parts per liter of air.

PVC: Polyvinyl Chloride is a plastic material that is used for many purposes such as rigid plastic pipes, thin food wrapping, clothing, and shoes, to name a few.

Surfactant: a chemical that breaks down the surface tension of a liquid, allowing it to either foam or penetrate solids.

Tannin: These are naturally occurring compounds that are found in plants. They have an astringent or drying effect. Some of the foods you may recognise them in are black tea, dark chocolate, and wine and they account for the bitter taste.

TDCPP (Chlorinated Tris): is a Chlorophosphate that is used as a fire retardant and plasticizer in various plastic foams, resins, and latexes. It was used as a flame retardant in automobile and truck upholstery, draperies, wall coverings, and in children's and infant's sleepwear.

TEA (triethanolamine): is produced by combining ethylene oxide with ammonia. It is used as a buffering agent, masking and fragrance ingredient, and a surfactant, however, its primary use as a pH adjuster. It may cause skin and eye irritation.

Toluene: a colorless, water-insoluble, flammable liquid, made from coal tar and petroleum. It is used in the manufacture of benzoic acid, benzaldehyde, TNT, and other organic compounds.

Trichloroethylene: most often used as a degreasing agent for metals and as a solvent for fats, oils, and waxes.

Triglyceride: Triglycerides are a type of fat (lipid) found in your blood that store unused calories. Having high levels of these triglycerides in your body can increase your risk of heart disease.

UVA: ultraviolet spectrum is nearest to visible light and extends from about 10 to 400 nm in wavelength. This radiation is present in sunlight, and causes tanning, damage, and aging to skin.

UVB (type B ultraviolet): This wave of radiation is also found in sunlight, has a wavelength between 290 and 320 nanometers, and can cause damage to the skin. Unlike UVA however, UVB rays cannot penetrate glass.

UVC: Ultraviolet light with wavelengths between 200–280 nanometers (nm). Often used as a disinfection method due to its ability to kill or inactivate microorganisms by breaking down nucleic acids and disrupting their DNA.

VOC-free: VOCs, or volatile organic compounds, are organic chemical compounds that evaporate under normal indoor temperature and pressure conditions. They are emitted as gases, or "off-gassed," and include a range of chemicals that may have short- or long-term adverse health effects. If a product is VOC-free, it does not contain these chemicals.

Xylene: Any of three oily, colorless, water-insoluble, flammable, toxic, isomeric liquids produced mainly from coal tar that is often used in the manufacture of dyes.

GLOSSARY OF TOXIC CHEMICALS TO AVOID

Atrazine: Atrazine is a commonly used herbicide on corn crops in the United States and is linked to reproductive issues as well as kidney, heart, and liver damage.[312]

Coal Tar: Also known as coal tar solution, tar, coal, carbo-cort, coal tar solution USP, crude coal tar, estar, impervotar, KC 261, larvitar, picis carbonis, naphtha, high solvent naphtha, naphtha distillate, benzin B70, and petroleum benzine. Found in shampoos and scalp treatments, soaps, hair dyes, and lotions. Studies have found that exposure to and application of coal tar produces skin tumors in mice. High exposure to coal tar has also been associated with cancer of the lung, bladder, kidney, and digestive tract.[313]

Dioxin: Dioxins are carcinogens that build up in the body as well as the food chain. They have also been linked to health effects of the immune and reproductive systems.[314]

Ethanolamines: Also known as Triethanolamine, diethanolamine, DEA, TEA, cocamide DEA, cocamide MEA, DEA-cetyl phosphate, DEA oleth-3 phosphate, lauramide DEA, linoleamide MEA, myristamide DEA, oleamide DEA, stearamide MEA, and TEA-lauryl sulfate. Found in soaps, shampoos, hair conditioners and dyes, lotions, shaving creams, paraffin and waxes, household cleaning products, pharmaceutical ointments, cosmetic products, fragrances, and sunscreens. Health concerns include damage to the liver and kidneys, environmental concerns (bioaccumulation), and organ system toxicity.[315]

Formaldehyde: Formaldehyde is considered a known human carcinogen by many experts and government bodies, including the United States National Toxicology Program.[316] Look for the following forms of the toxic substance on the ingredients list: formaldehyde, DMDM hydantoin, imidazolidinyl urea, diazolidinyl urea, quaternium-15 polyoxymethylene urea, sodium hydroxymethylglycinate, 2-bromo-2-nitropropane-1, 3-diol (bronopol) and glyoxal. Found in nail polish, nail glue, eyelash glue, hair gel, hair-smoothing products, shampoo, body wash, and color cosmetics.[317]

Glycol Ethers: Also known as 2-butoxyethanol (EGBE) and methoxydiglycol (DEGME). They are common solvents found in paints, cleaning products, brake fluid, and cosmetics. The European Union says that some of these chemicals "may damage fertility or the unborn child." Studies of painters have linked exposure to certain glycol ethers to blood abnormalities and lower sperm counts.[318]

Parabens: Also known as ethylparaben, butylparaben, methylparaben, propylparaben, isobutylparaben, isopropylparaben, and basically anything ending in paraben. Found in shampoos, conditioners, lotions, facial and shower cleansers, and scrubs. Parabens can act as estrogens and disrupt hormone signaling and may possibly be linked to breast cancer.[319]

Perchlorate: perchlorate, a component in rocket fuel, has been found in the U.S. in some produce and milk.[320] It has been linked, though not conclusively, to disrupt the thyroid hormone balance that regulates metabolism in adults and are critical for proper brain and organ development in infants and young children.[321]

Phthalates: Also known as phthalate, DEP, DBP, DEHP, and fragrance in labeling. Found in color cosmetics, fragranced lotions, body washes, hair care products, and nail polish. Scientific studies link phthalate exposure to reproductive abnormalities and endocrine disruption.[322]

Polyacrylamide: Also known as polyacrylamide; acrylamide; polyacrylate, polyquaternium, acrylate. Found in facial moisturizers, anti-aging products, color cosmetics, lotions, hair products, sunscreens, and many personal care products. Health concerns are that polyacrylamide can break down into acrylamide, which is a carcinogen. Reproductive and developmental toxicity are also a possibility.[323]

Perfluorooctanoic acid (PFOA): Found in Foundation, pressed powder, loose powder, bronzer, blush, eye shadow, mascara, shave gel, lip balm, anti-aging lotion, and non-stick cookware. In mice it has been shown to cause delayed reproductive development.[324]

Resorcinol: Also known as 1,3-benzenediol, resorcin, 1,3-dihydroxybenzene (m-hydroxybenzyl, m-dihydroxyphenol). Found in hair dyes, shampoos/hair lotions, peels, and in products used to treat acne, eczema, and other dermatological issues. Health concerns include skin and eye irritant, skin sensitizer, organ system toxicity, and possible endocrine disrupting chemical (EDC).[325]

Sodium Lauryl Sulfate/ Sodium Laureth Sulfate (SLS): Found in many personal hygiene products such as shampoos, toothpastes, mouthwashes, body wash, soaps, and detergents. If improperly diluted SLS can cause skin and eye irritation, and damage or even blindness at higher concentrations.[326]

Triclosan: Also known as triclosan (TSC) and triclocarban (TCC). Found in antibacterial soaps and detergents, tooth whitening products, antiperspirants/deodorants, shaving creams, and certain cosmetics. Health concerns include endocrine disruption, triclosan-resistant bacteria, and environmental toxicity.[327]

CITATIONS

1. Stemp-Morlock G. (2008). Mercury: cleanup for broken CFLs. *Environmental health perspectives*, 116(9), A378.

2. Nicole, Wendee. "Ultraviolet Leaks from CFLs." *Environmental Health Perspectives*, National Institute of Environmental Health Sciences, Oct. 2012, ncbi.nlm.nih.gov/pmc/articles/PMC3491932/.

3. Jaadane I., Boulenguez P., Chahory S., Carré S., Savoldelli M., Jonet L., Behar-Cohen F., Martinsons C., Torriglia A. (2015). Retinal damage induced by commercial light emitting diodes (LEDs). *Free Radical Biology and Medicine*, 84:373-384. doi: 10.1016/j.freeradbiomed.2015.03.034

4. Babrauskas, V., Blum, A., Daley R. and Birnbaum L., 2011. Flame Retardants in Furniture Foam: Benefits and Risks. Fire Safety Science 10: 265-278. 10.3801/IAFSS.FSS.10-265

5. U.S. Environmental Protection Agency. 1987. The total exposure assessment methodology (TEAM) study: Summary and analysis. EPA/600/6-87/002a. Washington, DC.

6. Kim, Sanghwa, et al. "Characterization of Air Freshener Emission: the Potential Health Effects." The Journal of Toxicological Sciences (J. Toxicol. Sci.), vol. 40, no. 5, 3 June 2015, pp. 535–547. JSTOR, jstage.jst.go.jp/article/jts/40/5/40_535/_pdf.

7. Steinemann, Anne. "Fragranced Consumer Products: Exposures and Effects from Emissions." *Air Quality, Atmosphere, & Health*, Springer Netherlands, 2016, ncbi.nlm.nih.gov/pmc/articles/PMC5093181/.

8. nrdc.org/media/2007/070919September 19, 2007. "New Study: Common Air Fresheners Contain Chemicals That May Affect Human Reproductive Development." *NRDC*, 4 May 2017, nrdc.org/media/2007/070919.

9. Fisher, B. E. "Scents and Sensitivity." Environmental Health Perspectives, vol. 106, no. 12, Dec. 1998, pp. 594–599.

10. La Merrill, Michelle, et al. "Toxicological Function of Adipose Tissue: Focus on Persistent Organic Pollutants." Environmental Health Perspectives, vol. 121, no. 2, Feb. 2013, pp. 162–167.

11. "1,4-Dichlorobenzene." *National Center for Biotechnology Information. PubChem Compound Database*, U.S. National Library of Medicine, 2005, pubchem.ncbi.nlm.nih.gov/compound/4685#section=Use-and-Manufacturing.

12. "Orange Essential Oil May Help Alleviate Post-Traumatic Stress Disorder." *ScienceDaily*, ScienceDaily, 24 Apr. 2017, sciencedaily.com/releases/2017/04/170424141354.htm.

13. Shah, G., Shri, R., Panchal, V., Sharma, N., Singh, B., & Mann, A. S. (2011). Scientific basis for the therapeutic use of Cymbopogon citratus, stapf (Lemon grass). Journal of advanced pharmaceutical technology & research, 2(1), 3–8. doi:10.4103/2231-4040.79796

14. Inglezakis, Vassilis J. "Zeolites in Soil Remediation Processes." Handbook of Natural Zeolites, Bentham Science Publishers, 2012, pp. 545–562.

15. United States, Congress, Research and Development, and E. Timothy Oppelt. "Candles and Incense as Potential Sources of Indoor Pollution." National Risk Management, 2001, pp. 1–53.

16. DOL. "Health Hazards and Protective Measures." United States Department of Labor, 2020, osha.gov/SLTC/toluene/ health_hazards.htmlemergency.cdc.gov/agent/benzene/basics/facts.asp.

17. United States Environmental Protection Agency. (2015). List of Lists: Consolidated List of Chemicals Subject to the Emergency Planning and Community Right To-Know Act (EPCRA), Comprehensive Environmental Response, Compensation and Liability Act (CERCLA) and Section 112(r) of the Clean Air Act. epa.gov/emergencies: Office of Solid Waste and Emergency Response.

18. Becher, Rune, and Johan Øvrevik. "Do Carpets Impair Indoor Air Quality and Cause Adverse Health Outcomes: A Review." Int J Environ Res Public Health, Feb. 2018, ncbi.nlm.nih.gov/pmc/articles/PMC585

19. Solet, David, et al. "Perchloroethylene Exposure Assessment Among Dry Cleaning Workers." American Industrial Hygiene Association Journal, 51:10, 566-574, 1990, DOI: 10.1080/15298669091370112

20. United States, Congress, National Health and Environmental Effects Research Laboratory, and Daniele Wikoff. "Human Health Effects of Brominated Flame Retardants." vol. 69, Organohalogen Compounds, 2007, pp. 670–67

21. Lam, Juleen, et al. "Developmental PBDE Exposure and IQ/ADHD in Childhood: A Systematic Review and Meta-Analysis." Environmental Health Perspectives, vol. 125, no. 8, 2017, pp. 086001-1-086001-17., doi:10.1289/ehp1632.

22. Tickner, Joel, and Yvie Torrie. "Presumption of Safety: Limits of Federal Policies on Toxic Substances in Consumer Products." Lowell Center for Sustainable Production , 2008, pp. 02-20.

23. Callahan, Patricia, and Sam Roe. "Fear Fans Flames for Chemical Makers." Chicago Tribune, 6 May 2012.

24. foam.pratt.duke.edu/ "How Does the Duke University Foam Project Work?" How Does the Duke University Foam Project Work? | Superfund Analytical Chemistry Core, foam.pratt.duke.edu

25. United States, Congress, ATSDR. "Public Health Statement for Nitrobenzene." Public Health Statement for Nitrobenzene, Agency for Toxic Substances and Disease Registry, 2020.

26. Ouyang, Jenny. "Hormonally Mediated Effects of Artificial Light at Night on Behavior and Fitness: Linking Endocrine Mechanisms with Function." Journal of Experimental Biology, 15 Mar. 2018, doi:10.1242/jeb.156893.

27. SCENIHR (Scientific Committee on Emerging and Newly Identified Health Risks). (2012, March 19). *Health Effects of Artificial Light.* Retrieved from: ec.europa.eu/health/scientific_committees/emerging/docs/scenihr_o_035.pdf

28. Joseph, A., Ph.D. (2006). Impact of Light on Outcomes in Healthcare Settings. *The Center for Health Design.*

29. Kuse, Y., Ogawa, K., Tsuruma, K., Shimazawa, M., & Hara, H. (2014). Damage of photoreceptor-derived cells in culture induced by light emitting diode-derived blue light. Scientific Reports, 4(1). doi:10.1038/srep05223

30. Oh, Ji Hye, et al. "Healthy, Natural, Efficient and Tunable Lighting: Four-Package White LEDs for Optimizing the Circadian Effect, Color Quality and Vision Performance." Nature, 2014, pp. 1–9., doi:10.1038/lsa.2014.22.

31. Foverskov, Melinda. "The Ultimate Guide To Red Light Therapy And Near-Infrared Light Therapy (Updated 2018)." *The Energy Blueprint,* The Energy Blueprint, 29 Dec. 2019, theenergyblueprint.com/red-light-therapy-ultimate-guide/.

32. Fernanda Guanipa, Maria. "Sick Building Syndrome Can Be Produced by Wallpaper Fungi." *Pulse Headlines,* 24 June 2017, pulseheadlines.com/sick-building-syndrome-produced-wallpaper-fungi/64535/.

33. Carroll, Linda. "Chemicals in Vinyl Flooring and Wallpaper Raise Worries." *NBCNews.com,* NBCUniversal News Group, 22 Nov. 2010, nbcnews.com/id/39728598/ns/health-childrens_health/t/chemicals-vinyl-flooring-wallpaper-raise-worries/.

34. Brankica Aleksic, Marjorie Draghi, Sebastien Ritoux, Sylviane Bailly, Marlène Lacroix, Isabelle P. Oswald, Jean-Denis Bailly, Enric Robine. Aerosolization of Mycotoxins after Growth of Toxinogenic Fungi on Wallpaper. Applied & Environmental Microbiology. Aug 2017, 83 (16) e01001-17; DOI: 10.1128/AEM.01001-17

35. "Ionization vs Photoelectric." *Ionization vs Photoelectric,* National Fire Protection Association, nfpa.org/Public-Education/ Staying-safe/Safety-equipment/Smoke-alarms/Ionization-vs-photoelectric.

36. Agency for Toxic Substances and Disease Registry (ATSDR). 2001. *Toxicological profile for Asbestos.* Atlanta, GA: U.S. Department of Health and Human Services, Public Health Service.

37. "When Is Asbestos Dangerous?" *Environmental Health and Safety,* 21 July 2009, ehs.oregonstate.edu/asb-when.

38. "Health Risks of an Inactive Lifestyle." *MedlinePlus,* U.S. National Library of Medicine, 9 Jan. 2020, medlineplus.gov/ healthrisksofaninactivelifestyle.html.

39. J Lennert Veerman, Genevieve N Healy, Linda J Cobiac, Theo Vos, Elisabeth A H Winkler, Neville Owen, David W Dunstan. (2012, December 1). Television viewing time and reduced life expectancy: a life table analysis. *British Journal of Sports Medicine.* 46:927-930.

40. Department of Health & Human Services. "Exercise and Mood." *Better Health Channel,* Department of Health & Human Services, 24 Jan. 2018, betterhealth.vic.gov.au/health/healthyliving/exercise-and-mood.

41. Wolverton, B.C., and Anne Johnson. "Interior Landscape Plants for Indoor Air Pollution Abatement." NASA Technical Reports Server, 15 Sept. 1989, ntrs.nasa.gov/archive/nasa/casi.ntrs.nasa.gov/19930073077.pdf.

42. Cullen, Lindsy. "Plants Used By NASA to Protect You From Deadly Airborne Chemicals." *BillyOh,* Kybotech Limited, 19 Apr. 2018, billyoh.com/extra/blog/garden/chemical-protective-plants/.

43. "Dioxin." *Dioxin,* Illinois Department of Public Health, idph.state.il.us/cancer/factsheets/dioxin.htm.

44. "Toxic Substances Portal—Sulfur Trioxide & Sulfuric Acid." *Centers for Disease Control and Prevention,* Centers for Disease Control and Prevention, 21 Jan. 2015, atsdr.cdc.gov/phs/phs.asp?id=254&tid=47.

45. Roeder, Amy. "Harmful, Untested Chemicals Rife in Personal Care Products." *News,* The President and Fellows of Harvard College, 19 Feb. 2014, hsph.harvard.edu/news/features/harmful-chemicals-in-personal-care-products/.

46. Nevin, K C, and T Rajamohan. "Effect of Topical Application of Virgin Coconut Oil on Skin Components and Antioxidant Status during Dermal Wound Healing in Young Rats." *Skin Pharmacology and Physiology,* U.S. National Library of Medicine, 3 June 2010, ncbi.nlm.nih.gov/pubmed/20523108.

47. Intahphuak, S, et al. "Anti-Inflammatory, Analgesic, and Antipyretic Activities of Virgin Coconut Oil." *Pharmaceutical Biology,* U.S. National Library of Medicine, Feb. 2010, ncbi.nlm.nih.gov/pubmed/20645831.

48. Yagnik, Darshna, et al. "Antimicrobial Activity of Apple Cider Vinegar against Escherichia Coli, Staphylococcus Aureus and Candida Albicans; Downregulating Cytokine and Microbial Protein Expression." *Scientific Reports,* Nature Publishing Group UK, 29 Jan. 2018, ncbi.nlm.nih.gov/pmc/articles/PMC5788933/.

49. GESAMP (Joint Group of Experts on the Scientific Aspects of Marine Environmental Protection). (2015). *Sources, Fate, and Effects of Microplastics in the Marine Environment: A Global Assessment.*

50. Smith, Madeleine, et al. "Microplastics in Seafood and the Implications for Human Health." *Current Environmental Health Reports,* Springer International Publishing, Sept. 2018, ncbi.nlm.nih.gov/pmc/articles/PMC6132564/.

51. Anthony, Kiara. "Baking Soda and Acne: Benefits, Risk, and Treatment Methods." Healthline.com, 27 Mar. 2019, healthline.com/health/baking-soda-acne.

52. Choi, Hyeon-Son, et al. "Topical Application of Spent Coffee Ground Extracts Protects Skin from Ultraviolet B-Induced Photoaging in Hairless Mice." *Photochemical & Photobiological Sciences*, The Royal Society of Chemistry, 10 May 2016, pubs. rsc.org/en/content/articlelanding/2016/PP/C6PP00045B#!divAbstract.

53. "The Benefits and Risks of Dry Brushing." *Healthline*, Healthline Media, healthline.com/health/dry-brushing#benefits.

54. Engeli, Roger T, et al. "Interference of Paraben Compounds with Estrogen Metabolism by Inhibition of 17β-Hydroxysteroid Dehydrogenases." *International Journal of Molecular Sciences*, MDPI, 19 Sept. 2017, ncbi.nlm.nih.gov/pmc/articles/ PMC5618656/.

55. United States, Congress, National Toxicology Program, and M.D. Boudreaux. "NTP Technical Report on the Photococarcinogenesis Study of Retinoic Acid and Retinyl Palmitate." National Institutes of Health Public Service, 2012, pp. 03–3557.

56. Kukreja, Kushneet. "How To Remove Excess Sebum From Scalp: Causes And Tips." *Oliva Skin & Hair Care Clinics*, Oliva Clinic, 16 Sept. 2019, olivaclinic.com/blog/sebum-on-scalp/.

57. "Dry Eyes." *Mayo Clinic*, Mayo Foundation for Medical Education and Research, 14 Mar. 2019, mayoclinic.org/diseases-conditions/dry-eyes/diagnosis-treatment/drc-20371869.

58. Saitta, Peter, et al. "Is There a True Concern Regarding the Use of Hair Dye and Malignancy Development?: a Review of the Epidemiological Evidence Relating Personal Hair Dye Use to the Risk of Malignancy." *The Journal of Clinical and Aesthetic Dermatology*, Matrix Medical Communications, Jan. 2013, ncbi.nlm.nih.gov/pmc/articles/PMC3543291/.

59. Ethanolamine Compounds (MEA, DEA, TEA And Others). (2013, November 5). The Campaign for Safe Cosmetics. Retrieved from safecosmetics.org/get-the-facts/chemicals-of-concern/ethanolamine-compounds

60. Whelan, Corey. "Hair Dye Allergy: Symptoms, Treatment and Color Alternatives." Healthline.com, 1 Mar. 2019, healthline.com/health/hair-dye-allergy.

61. Whelan, Corey. "Hair Dye Allergy: Symptoms, Treatment and Color Alternatives." Healthline.com, 1 Mar. 2019, healthline.com/health/hair-dye-allergy.

62. Lin, Tzu-Kai, et al. "Anti-Inflammatory and Skin Barrier Repair Effects of Topical Application of Some Plant Oils." *International Journal of Molecular Sciences*, MDPI, 27 Dec. 2017, ncbi.nlm.nih.gov/pmc/articles/ PMC5796020/#!po=42.7419/.

63. Mahmood, Khawaja Tahir. "Moringa Oleifera: a Natural Gift-A Review." Journal of Pharmaceutical Sciences and Research, vol. 2, 2010.

64. "Triphenyl Phosphate." *National Center for Biotechnology Information. PubChem Compound Database*, U.S. National Library of Medicine, pubchem.ncbi.nlm.nih.gov/compound/Triphenyl-phosphate#section=Toxicity-Summary.

65. Mendelsohn, Emma. "Nail Polish as a Source of Exposure to Triphenyl Phosphate." Environment International, Jan. 2016, pp. 45–51., doi:10.1016/j.envint.2015.10.005.

66. Mendelsohn, Emma. "Nail Polish as a Source of Exposure to Triphenyl Phosphate." Environment International, Jan. 2016, pp. 45–51., doi:10.1016/j.envint.2015.10.005.

67. "TPHP: a New Endocrine Disruptor." *EWG*, 19 Oct. 2015, ewg.org/research/nailed/tphp-new-endocrine-disruptor.

68. Kearney, Caitlin. "Why I Smell Like It's 1903." National Museum of American History, 10 Nov. 2014, americanhistory. si.edu/ar/blog/2014/09/why-i-smell-like-its-1903.html.

69. Urban1, Julie, et al. "The Effect of Habitual and Experimental Antiperspirant and Deodorant Product Use on the Armpit Microbiome." *PeerJ*, PeerJ Inc., 2 Feb. 2016, peerj.com/articles/1605.

70. Oatman-Stanford, Hunter. "A Brief History of Body Odor." *The Week—All You Need to Know about Everything That Matters*, The Week, 27 Mar. 2016, theweek.com/articles/614722/brief-history-body-odor.

71. Ngan, Vanessa. "Antiperspirant." *Antiperspirant | DermNet NZ*, 2005, dermnetnz.org/topics/antiperspirant/.

72. Sears, M. E., Kerr, K. J., & Bray, R. I. (2012). Arsenic, cadmium, lead, and mercury in sweat: a systematic review. *Journal of environmental and public health*, 2012, 184745. doi:10.1155/2012/184745

73. Darbre, P. (2005). Aluminium, antiperspirants and breast cancer. *Journal of Inorganic Biochemistry*,99(9), 1912-1919. doi:10.1016/j.jinorgbio.2005.06.001

74. Farasani, A, and P D Darbre. "Effects of Aluminium Chloride and Aluminium Chlorohydrate on DNA Repair in MCF10A Immortalised Non-Transformed Human Breast Epithelial Cells." *Journal of Inorganic Biochemistry*, U.S. National Library of Medicine, Nov. 2015, ncbi.nlm.nih.gov/pubmed/26319584.

75. Engeli, Roger T, et al. "Interference of Paraben Compounds with Estrogen Metabolism by Inhibition of 17β-Hydroxysteroid Dehydrogenases." *International Journal of Molecular Sciences*, MDPI, 19 Sept. 2017, ncbi.nlm.nih.gov/pmc/articles/ PMC5618656/.

76. Colombo, P. "Buccal Drug Administration." *Buccal Drug Administration—an Overview | ScienceDirect Topics*, 2007, sciencedirect.com/topics/medicine-and-dentistry/buccal-drug-administration.

77. Tobacman, J K. "Review of Harmful Gastrointestinal Effects of Carrageenan in Animal Experiments." *Environmental Health Perspectives*, U.S. National Library of Medicine, Oct. 2001, ncbi.nlm.nih.gov/pmc/articles/PMC1242073/.

78. Weatherly, Lisa M, and Julie A Gosse. "Triclosan Exposure, Transformation, and Human Health Effects." *Journal of Toxicology and Environmental Health. Part B, Critical Reviews*, U.S. National Library of Medicine, 2017, ncbi.nlm.nih.gov/pmc/articles/PMC6126357/.

79. "Environmental Health and Medicine Education." *Centers for Disease Control and Prevention*, Centers for Disease Control and Prevention, 2007, atsdr.cdc.gov/csem/csem.asp?csem=12&po=14.

80. Shanbhag, Vagish Kumar L. "Oil Pulling for Maintaining Oral Hygiene—A Review." *Journal of Traditional and Complementary Medicine*, Elsevier, 6 June 2016, ncbi.nlm.nih.gov/pmc/articles/PMC5198813/.

81. Dentist.net. "XYLITOL and YOUR TEETH by Dentist.net." *Dentist.net*, Dentist.net, 2020, dentist.net/pages/xylitol-teeth.

82. Kleber, C J, et al. "Laboratory Assessment of Tooth Whitening by Sodium Bicarbonate Dentifrices." *The Journal of Clinical Dentistry*, U.S. National Library of Medicine, 1998, ncbi.nlm.nih.gov/pubmed/10518866.

83. Nordqvist, Christian. "Coconut Oil May Prevent Tooth Decay." *Medical News Today*, MediLexicon International, 4 Sept. 2012, medicalnewstoday.com/articles/249804.php#1.

84. Ghadimi, Elnaz, et al. "Trace Elements Can Influence the Physical Properties of Tooth Enamel." *SpringerPlus*, Springer International Publishing, 2 Oct. 2013, ncbi.nlm.nih.gov/pmc/articles/PMC3795877/.

85. Moosavi, Maryam. "Bentonite Clay as a Natural Remedy: A Brief Review." Iranian journal of public health vol. 46, 9 (2017): 1176-1183.

86. Sudharsana, A. "Tooth Friendly Chocolate." Journal of Pharmaceutical Sciences and Research, vol. 7, 2015, pp. 49–50.

87. Webster, Glenys. "Potential Human Health Effects of Perfluorinated Chemicals." National Collaborating Centre for Environmental Health, 2010, ncceh.ca/sites/default/files/Health_effects_PFCs_Oct_2010.pdf

88. Van Dieren, S. "Coffee and Tea Consumption and Risk of Type 2 Diabetes." Diabetologia, Sept. 2009, doi:10.1007/s00125-009-1516-3.

89. "Talcum Powder and Cancer." *American Cancer Society*, American Cancer Society, 2020, cancer.org/cancer/cancer-causes/talcum-powder-and-cancer.html.

90. Jiang-nan Wu, Suzanne C Ho, Chun Zhou, Wen-hua Ling, Wei-qing Chen, Cui-ling Wang, Yu-ming Chen. (2009, December). Coffee consumption and risk of coronary heart diseases: A meta-analysis of 21 prospective cohort studies. *International Journal of Cardiology*. doi.org/10.1016/j.ijcard.2008.06.051

91. Isle, Jay W. Belle, et al. "American Pediatric Association Recommends against Using Baby Powder." *Legal Reader*, 18 Sept. 2017, legalreader.com/american-pediatric-association-recommends-against-using-baby-powder/.

92. Pavey, Sandra. "Sun Damage and Cancer: How UV Radiation Affects Our Skin." *Diamantina Institute*, The University of Queensland Australia, 6 Feb. 2017, di.uq.edu.au/article/2017/02/sun-damage-and-cancer-how-uv-radiation-affects-our-skin.

93. Schuch, André Passaglia, et al. "Sunlight Damage to Cellular DNA: Focus on Oxidatively Generated Lesions." *Free Radical Biology and Medicine*, Pergamon, 18 Jan. 2017, sciencedirect.com/science/article/pii/S0891584917300382.

94. "EWG's 2019 Guide to Safer Sunscreens." *EWG*, Environmental Working Group, 2020, ewg.org/sunscreen/report/nanoparticles-in-sunscreen/.

95. Korać, Radava R, and Kapil M Khambholja. "Potential of Herbs in Skin Protection from Ultraviolet Radiation." *Pharmacognosy Reviews*, Medknow Publications & Media Pvt Ltd, July 2011, ncbi.nlm.nih.gov/pmc/articles/PMC3263051/.

96. Weatherly, Lisa M, and Julie A Gosse. "Triclosan Exposure, Transformation, and Human Health Effects." *Journal of Toxicology and Environmental Health. Part B, Critical Reviews*, U.S. National Library of Medicine, 2017, ncbi.nlm.nih.gov/pmc/articles/PMC6126357/.

97. Hormann, Annette M., et al. "Holding Thermal Receipt Paper and Eating Food after Using Hand Sanitizer Results in High Serum Bioactive and Urine Total Levels of Bisphenol A (BPA)." PLoS ONE, vol. 9, no. 10, 2014, doi:10.1371/journal.pone.0110509.

98. Suzuki M, Yamada K, Nagao M, et al. "Antimicrobial Ointments and Methicillin-Resistant Staphylococcus Aureus." Emerging Infectious Diseases, vol. 17, no. 10, Oct. 2011, doi:10.3201/eid1710.101365.

99. Niaz, Kamal, et al. "Health Benefits of Manuka Honey as an Essential Constituent for Tissue Regeneration." *Current Drug Metabolism*, U.S. National Library of Medicine, 2017, ncbi.nlm.nih.gov/pubmed/28901255.

100. Gotter, Ana. "8 Home Remedies for Hemorrhoids." Healthline.com, 2017, healthline.com/health/home-remedies-for-hemorrhoids.

101. Abdel-Rahman, A., et al. "Stress and Combined Exposure to Low Doses of Pyridostigmine Bromide, DEET, and Permethrin Produce Neurochemical and Neuropathological Alterations in Cerebral Cortex, Hippocampus, and Cerebellum." Journal of toxicology and environmental health, 2004, 163-92. 10.1080/15287390490264802.

102. Abou-Donia, Mohamed B, et al. "Co-Exposure to Pyridostigmine Bromide, DEET, and/or Permethrin Causes Sensorimotor Deficit and Alterations in Brain Acetylcholinesterase Activity." Pharmacology Biochemistry and Behavior, Elsevier, 19 Dec. 2003, sciencedirect.com/science/article/pii/S0091305703003459.

103. "Catnip Repels Mosquitoes More Effectively Than DEET." ScienceDaily, ScienceDaily, 28 Aug. 2001, sciencedaily.com/releases/2001/08/010828075659.htm.

104. Center for Devices and Radiological Health. "Menstrual Tampons and Pads: Information for Premarket Guidance." U.S. Food and Drug Administration, FDA, fda.gov/regulatory-information/search-fda-guidance-documents/menstrual-tampons-and-pads-information-premarket-notification-submissions-510ks-guidance-industry.

105. Stone, Janis, and Wendy Wintersteen. "Learn About Pesticides and Clothes." NASD, Iowa State University , 1992, nasdonline.org/1254/d001058/learn-about-pesticides-and-clothes.html.

106. Burns, Carla, and Kali Rauhe. "Study: Elevated Levels of Toxic Chemicals Found in Menstrual Pads and Disposable Diapers." EWG, 2019, ewg.org/news-and-analysis/2019/03/study-elevated-levels-toxic-chemicals-found-menstrual-pads-and-disposable.

107. Burns, Carla, and Kali Rauhe. "Study: Elevated Levels of Toxic Chemicals Found in Menstrual Pads and Disposable Diapers." EWG, 2019, ewg.org/news-and-analysis/2019/03/study-elevated-levels-toxic-chemicals-found-menstrual-pads-and-disposable.

108. Burns, Carla, and Kali Rauhe. "Study: Elevated Levels of Toxic Chemicals Found in Menstrual Pads and Disposable Diapers." EWG, 2019, ewg.org/news-and-analysis/2019/03/study-elevated-levels-toxic-chemicals-found-menstrual-pads-and-disposable.

109. Rabago, David, et al. "Efficacy of Daily Hypertonic Saline Nasal Irrigation among Patients with Sinusitis: a Randomized Controlled Trial." The Journal of Family Practice, U.S. National Library of Medicine, Dec. 2002, ncbi.nlm.nih.gov/pubmed/12540331.

110. Asha'ari, Zamzil Amin, et al. "Ingestion of Honey Improves the Symptoms of Allergic Rhinitis: Evidence from a Randomized Placebo-Controlled Trial in the East Coast of Peninsular Malaysia." Annals of Saudi Medicine, King Faisal Specialist Hospital and Research Centre, 2013, ncbi.nlm.nih.gov/pubmed/24188941.

111. Asha'ari, Zamzil Amin, et al. "Ingestion of Honey Improves the Symptoms of Allergic Rhinitis: Evidence from a Randomized Placebo-Controlled Trial in the East Coast of Peninsular Malaysia." Annals of Saudi Medicine, King Faisal Specialist Hospital and Research Centre, 2013, ncbi.nlm.nih.gov/pmc/articles/PMC6074882/.

112. Johri, et al. "Anti-Allergic Effects of Herbal Product from Allium Cepa (Bulb)." Mary Ann Liebert, Inc., Publishers, 21 May 2009, liebertpub.com/doi/abs/10.1089/jmf.2007.0642.

113. "Allergies." Liver Doctor, liverdoctor.com/allergies/.

114. "Signs Your Liver Needs A Detox." Quicksilver Scientific, 12 Sept. 2019, quicksilverscientific.com/blog/signs-your-liver-needs-a-detox/.

115. Elbossaty, Walaa Fikry. "Pharmaceutical Influences of Epsom Salts." American Journal of Pharmacology and Pharmacotherapeutics, IMedPub, 31 July 2018, imedpub.com/articles/pharmaceutical-influences-of-epsom-salts.php?aid=23254.

116. de Baaij, Jeroen H F, et al. "Magnesium in Man: Implications for Health and Disease." Physiological Reviews, U.S. National Library of Medicine, Jan. 2015, ncbi.nlm.nih.gov/pubmed/25540137.

117. Strott, Charles A. "Sulfonation and Molecular Action." Endocrine Reviews, U.S. National Library of Medicine, Oct. 2002, ncbi.nlm.nih.gov/pubmed/12372849.

118. Nordqvist, Joseph. "The Health Benefits of Eucalyptus." Medical News Today, Jan. 2018, medicalnewstoday.com/articles/26658

119. Schutes, Jade. "The Quality of Essential Oils." National Association for Holistic Therapy, naha.org/assets/uploads/The_Quality_of_Essential_Oils_Journal.pdf.

120. Messoud, Hnia Chograni Chokri. "Comparative Chemical Composition and Antibacterial Activities of Myrtus Communis L. Essential Oils Isolated from Tunisian and Algerian Population." Journal of Plant Pathology & Microbiology, vol. 04, no. 07, 2013, doi:10.4172/2157-7471.1000186.

121. Alipour, Ghazal, et al. "Review of Pharmacological Effects of Myrtus communis L. and its Active Constituents." Journal of Phytotherapy Research, 2014, PTR. 28. 10.1002/ptr.5122.

122. "Myrrh." The Free Dictionary, Farlex, encyclopedia2.thefreedictionary.com/myrrh.

123. Harvard Health Publishing. "Blue Light Has a Dark Side." *Harvard Health*, 2012, health.harvard.edu/staying-healthy/blue-light-has-a-dark-side.

124. Dubocovich, Margarita L, and Magdalena Markowska. "Functional MT1 and MT2 Melatonin Receptors in Mammals." *Endocrine*, U.S. National Library of Medicine, July 2005, ncbi.nlm.nih.gov/pubmed/16217123.

125. Zhao, J., Tian, Y., Nie , J., Xu, J., & Liu, D. (2012). Red Light and the Sleep Quality and Endurance Performance of Chinese Female Basketball Players. Retrieved from ncbi.nlm.nih.gov/pmc/articles/PMC3499892/

126. Komori , T., Matsumoto, T., Motomura, E., & Shiroyama, T. (2006). The sleep-enhancing effect of valerian inhalation and sleep-shortening effect of lemon inhalation. Retrieved from ncbi.nlm.nih.gov/pubmed/16857858

127. Koulivand, P. H., Ghadiri, M. K., & Gorji, A. Lavender and the Nervous System. Retrieved from ncbi.nlm.nih.gov/pmc/articles/PMC3612440/

128. Raudenbush, B., Koon, J., Smith, J., & Zoladz, P. (2003). Effects of Odorant Administration on Objective and Subjective Measures of Sleep Quality, Post-Sleep Mood and Alertness, and Cognitive Performance. *North American Journal of Psychology*, 5(2), 181-192.

129. Messoud, Hnia Chograni Chokri. "Comparative Chemical Composition and Antibacterial Activities of Myrtus Communis L. Essential Oils Isolated from Tunisian and Algerian Population." Journal of Plant Pathology & Microbiology, vol. 04, no. 07, 2013, doi:10.4172/2157-7471.1000186.

130. Jaakkola, Jouni J K, and Trudy L Knight. "The Role of Exposure to Phthalates from Polyvinyl Chloride Products in the Development of Asthma and Allergies: a Systematic Review and Meta-Analysis." *Environmental Health Perspectives*, National Institute of Environmental Health Sciences, July 2008, ncbi.nlm.nih.gov/pubmed/18629304.

131. Miller, J. D. (1989). CDC—NIOSH Publications and Products—Carcinogenic Effects of Exposure to Propylene Oxide (89-111). Retrieved from cdc.gov/niosh/docs/89-111/

132. Kim , BN, SC Cho, Y Kim, MS Shin, HJ Yoo, JW Kim, YH Yang, HW Kim, SY Bhang, and YC Hong. "Phthalates Exposure and Attention-deficit/Hyperactivity Disorder in School-Age Children.", November 2009. ncbi.nlm.nih.gov/pubmed/19748073.

133. Xu, Ying. "More Regulation, Public Awareness Needed to End Toxic Chemicals in Crib Mattresses." News.utexas.edu, The University of Texas at Austin, 27 May 2014, news.utexas.edu/2014/05/27/more-regulation-public-awareness-needed-to-end-toxic-chemicals-in-crib-mattresses/.

134. Agency for Toxic Substances and Disease Registry (ATSDR). Toxicological Profile for Styrene. U.S. Public Health Service, U.S. Department of Health and Human Services, Atlanta, GA. 1992.

135. "UNITED STATES DEPARTMENT OF LABOR." Occupational Safety and Health Administration. osha.gov/SLTC/butadiene/healtheffects.html.

136. "Synthetic Latex." *Synthetic Latex—an Overview | ScienceDirect Topics*, sciencedirect.com/topics/engineering/synthetic-latex.

137. Brigden, Kevin, et al. "Hazardous Chemicals in Branded Textile Products on Sale in 27 Places during 2012." Greenpeace Research Laboratories, 2012, greenpeace.org/archive-international/Global/international/publications/toxics/Water%202012/TechnicalReport-06-2012.pdf.

138. "Putting the Brakes on Fast Fashion." UN Environment, Nov. 2018, unenvironment.org/news-and-stories/story/putting-brakes-fast-fashion.

139. Luongo, Giovanna. *Chemicals in Textiles. A Potential Source for Human Exposure and Environmental Pollution*. Master's thesis, Stockholm University, 2015. Stockholm: Publit, 2015.

140. Messinger, Leah. "How Your Clothes Are Poisoning Our Oceans and Food Supply." The Guardian. June 20, 2016. Accessed April 15, 2019. theguardian.com/environment/2016/jun/20/microfibers-plastic-pollution-oceans-patagonia-synthetic-clothes-microbeads.

141. Browne, Mark Anthony, Phillip Crump, Stewart J. Niven, Emma Teuten, Andrew Tonkin, Tamara Galloway, and Richard Thompson. "Accumulation of Microplastic on Shorelines Woldwide: Sources and Sinks." ACS Publications. 2011. pubs.acs.org/doi/abs/10.1021/es201811s.

142. Kover, Frank. *Preliminary Study of Selected Potential Environmental Contaminants—Optical Brighteners, Methyl Chloroform, Trichloroethylene, Tetrachloroethylene, Ion Exchange Resins, Final Report*. (July 1975) EPA.

143. "Genetically Modified Cotton, CBAN Factsheet." CBAN, Feb. 2013, cban.ca/gmos/products/on-the-market/cotton/Genetically-Modified-Cotton-CBAN-Factsheet/.

144. "Report on Tide Pods Detergent, Original." EWG.org, Environmental Working Group, 2020, ewg.org/guides/cleaners/6127-TidePodsDetergentOriginal.

145. Kessler, Rebecca. "Dryer Vents: an Overlooked Source of Pollution?" *Environmental Health Perspectives*, National Institute of Environmental Health Sciences, Nov. 2011, ncbi.nlm.nih.gov/pmc/articles/PMC3226517/#r9.

146. Alvarez, et al. "Chemical Emissions from Residential Dryer Vents during Use of Fragranced Laundry Products." *Air Quality, Atmosphere & Health*, Springer Netherlands, 1 Jan. 1999, link.springer.com/article/10.1007/s11869-011-0156-1.

147. Alvarez, et al. "Chemical Emissions from Residential Dryer Vents during Use of Fragranced Laundry Products." *Air Quality, Atmosphere & Health*, Springer Netherlands, 1 Jan. 1999, link.springer.com/article/10.1007/s11869-011-0156-1.

148. Arif, Ahmed A., and George L. Delclos. "Association between Cleaning-related Chemicals and Work-related Asthma and Asthma Symptoms among Healthcare Professionals." Occupational and Environmental Medicine. January 2012. ncbi.nlm.nih.gov/pubmed/21602538.

149. Peltier, Karen. "For Greener Laundry, Skip Optical Brighteners." The Spruce, The Spruce, 19 Oct. 2019, thespruce.com/optical-brighteners-chemicals-not-needed-1707025.

150. Anne, Leigh. "Optical Brighteners." O ECOTEXTILES, oecotextiles.wordpress.com/category/chemicals/optical-brighteners/.

151. Benzoni, Thomas, and Jason D. Hatcher. Bleach Toxicity. Des Moines University, 2019, Bleach Toxicity.

152. United States, Congress, National Cancer Institute, and Abby B. Sandler. "Reducing Environmental Cancer Risk: What We Can Do Now.", National Institutes of Health, 2010.

153. McDermott, Michael J. "Tetrachloroethylene (PCE, Perc) Levels in Residential Dry Cleaner Buildings in Diverse Communities in New York City." Environmental Health Perspectives, Oct. 2005.

154. Sherlach, Katy S., Alexander P. Gorka, Alexa Dantzler, and Paul D. Roepe. "Quantification of Perchloroethylene Residues in Dry-cleaned Fabrics." Environmental Toxicology and Chemistry. September 20, 2011. setac.onlinelibrary.wiley.com/doi/abs/10.1002/etc.665.

155. Shaw, Gina. "How Much Water Do You Need? Can You Drink Too Much?" WebMD. ebmd.com/diet/features/water-for-weight-loss-diet#1.

156. *EWG's Tap Water Database: State of American Drinking Water*. Environmental Working Group. Retrieved from ewg.org/tapwater/state-of-american-drinking-water.php.

157. "Occurrence and Potential Biological Effects of Amphetamine on Stream Communities." Sylvia S. Lee, Alexis M. Paspalof, Daniel D. Snow, Erinn K. Richmond, Emma J. Rosi-Marshall, and John J. Kelly. Environmental Science & Technology **2016** 50 (17), 9727-9735

158. Scheer, Roddy, and Doug Moss. "External Medicine: Discarded Drugs May Contaminate 40 Million Americans' Drinking Water." Scientific American, Scientific American, 16 Sept. 2011, scientificamerican.com/article/pharmaceuticals-in-the-water/.

159. Doheny, Kathleen. "Drugs in Our Drinking Water?" WebMD, 10 Mar. 2008, webmd.com/a-to-z-guides/features/drugs-in-our-drinking-water#1.

160. Feldscher, Karen, and Karen Feldscher. "Unsafe Levels of Toxic Chemicals Found in Drinking Water of 33 States." Harvard Gazette. January 30, 2017. news.harvard.edu/gazette/story/2016/08/unsafe-levels-of-toxic-chemicals-found-in-drinking-water-of-33-states/.

161. United States, Congress, NRMR. "Risk Assessment Evaluation for Concentrated Animal Feeding Operations." EPA, 2004.

162. Dreams, Common. "Report: 64% of Bottled Water Is Tap Water, Costs 2000x More." EcoWatch, EcoWatch, 18 Dec. 2019, ecowatch.com/bottled-water-sources-tap-2537510642.html.

163. Mason, Sherri, and Victoria Welch. Synthetic Polymer Contamination in Bottled Water. State University of NY at Freedonia.

164. Walker, Bill, and Wicitra Mahotama. "170 Million in U.S. Drink Radioactive Tap Water. Trump Nominee Faked Data to Hide Cancer Risk." EWG, 11 Jan. 2018, ewg.org/research/170-million-us-drink-radioactive-tap-water-trump-nominee-faked-data-hide-cancer-risk.

165. Watanabe F, Abe K, Fujita T, Goto M, Hiemori M, Nakano Y. "Effects of Microwave Heating on the Loss of Vitamin B(12) in Foods." J Agric Food Chem. 1998 Jan 19;46(1):206-210.

166. Harvard Health Publishing. "Is Plastic a Threat to Your Health?" Harvard Health, Dec. 2019, health.harvard.edu/staying-healthy/is-plastic-a-threat-to-your-health.

167. Ogidi, Muyiwa, et al. "A Follow-Up Study Health Risk Assessment of Heavy Metal Leachability from Household Cookwares." Journal of Food Science and Toxicology, IMedPub, 9 Nov. 2017, imedpub.com/articles/a-followup-study-health-risk-assessment-of-heavy-metal-leachability-from-household-cookwares.php?aid=21347.

168. "Teflon and Other Non-Stick Pans Kill Birds." EWG, 3 Apr. 2003, ewg.org/research/pfcs-global-contaminants/teflon-and-other-non-stick-pans-kill-birds.

169. Kamerud, Kristen, and Kevin Hobbie. "Stainless Steel Leaches Nickel and Chromium into Foods During Cooking." Journal of Agricultural and Food Chemistry, Jan. 2015.

170. Mirza, Ambreen. "Aluminium in Brain Tissue in Familial Alzheimer's Disease." Journal of Trace Elements in Medicine and Biology, 2016, doi: doi.org/10.1016/j.jtemb.2016.12.001.

171. Ohlsen, M.V. Kroger, T. Trugvason, L.H. Skibsted, and K.F. Michaelsen. "Release of Iron Into Foods Cooked in an Iron Pot: Effect of PH, Salt, and Organic Acids." 2002. img2.timg.co.il/forums/1_167440814.pdf.

172. Geerligs, PD, BJ Brabin, and AA Omari. "Food Prepared in Iron Cooking Pots As an Intervention for Reducing Iron Deficiency Anaemia in Developing Countries: A Systematic Review.", August 2003. ncbi.nlm.nih.gov/pubmed/12859709.

173. Fralick , Michael, Aaron Thompson, and Ophyr Mourad. "Lead Toxicity from Glazed Ceramic Cookware", December 6, 2016. ncbi.nlm.nih.gov/pmc/articles/PMC5135532/.

174. Yang, Chun Z., and Stuart Yaniger. "Most Plastic Products Release Estrogenic Chemicals: A Potential Health Problem That Can Be Solved." Environmental Health Perspectives, July 2011, doi: dx.doi.org/10.1289%2Fehp.1003220

175. Sondi, Ivan, and Branka Salopek-Sondi. "Silver Nanoparticles as Antimicrobial Agent: A Case Study on E. Coli as a Model for Gram-negative Bacteria." Journal of Colloid and Interface Science. July 01, 2004. ncbi.nlm.nih.gov/pubmed/15158396.

176. Jung, Woo Kyung, Hye Cheong Koo, Ki Woo Kim, Sook Shin, So Hyun Kim, and Yong Ho Park. "Antibacterial Activity and Mechanism of Action of the Silver Ion in Staphylococcus Aureus and Escherichia Coli." Applied and Environmental Microbiology. April 2008. ncbi.nlm.nih.gov/pmc/articles/PMC2292600/#r20.

177. CY, Chien, et al. High Melamine Migration in Daily-Use Melamine-Made Tableware. Journal of Hazardous Materials, 2011.

178. Ingelfinger, Julie R. "Melamine and the Global Implications of Food Contamination." New England Journal of Medicine, vol. 359, no. 26, 2008, pp. 2745–2748., doi:10.1056/nejmp0808410.

179. Center for Food Safety and Applied Nutrition. "Melamine in Tableware Questions and Answers." U.S. Food and Drug Administration, 2017, fda.gov/food/chemicals/melamine-tableware-questions-and-answers.

180. CDC. "Phthalates Factsheet." Centers for Disease Control and Prevention, Centers for Disease Control and Prevention, 7 Apr. 2017, cdc.gov/biomonitoring/Phthalates_FactSheet.html.

181. "Cleaner Ratings | Oven Cleaner." EWG. ewg.org/guides/subcategories/39-OvenCleaner#.Wotera6nGM8.

182. "Oven Cleaner Poisoning: MedlinePlus Medical Encyclopedia." MedlinePlus. medlineplus.gov/ency/article/002800.htm.

183. Tucker, Jennifer. "Certification of Organic Crop Container Systems ." Received by USDA-Accredited Certifying Agents, 1400 Independence Avenue, 3 June 2019, Washington, D.C.

184. ECFR—Code of Federal Regulations." Electronic Code of Federal Regulations (ECFR), 2 Mar. 2020, ecfr.gov/cgi-bin/text-idx?c=ecfr&SID=9874504b6f1025eb0e6b67cadf9d3b40&rgn=div6&view=text&node=7:3.1.1.9.32.7&idno=7#se7.3.205_1601.

185. Consumer Reports. "The Trouble With Labels Like 'Natural' and 'All Natural'." Consumer Reports, 16 Feb. 2016, consumerreports.org/food-safety/the-trouble-with-labels-like-natural-and-all-natural/.

186. Aubrey, Allison. "Reviving An Heirloom Corn That Packs More Flavor And Nutrition." NPR, NPR, 22 Aug. 2013, npr.org/sections/thesalt/2013/08/22/209844877/reviving-an-heirloom-corn-that-packs-more-flavor-and-nutrition.

187. I-Sis. "'Stunning' Difference of GM from Non-GM Corn." The Permaculture Research Institute, 22 Apr. 2013, permaculturenews.org/2013/04/22/stunning-difference-of-gm-from-non-gm-corn/.

188. Sofi, Francesco, et al. "Effect of Triticum Turgidum Subsp. Turanicum Wheat on Irritable Bowel Syndrome: a Double-Blinded Randomised Dietary Intervention Trial." The British Journal of Nutrition, Cambridge University Press, 14 June 2014, ncbi.nlm.nih.gov/pubmed/24521561?dopt=Citation.

189. Kubsad, Deepika, et al. "Assessment of Glyphosate Induced Epigenetic Transgenerational Inheritance of Pathologies and Sperm Epimutations: Generational Toxicology." Scientific Reports, vol. 9, no. 1, 2019, doi:10.1038/s41598-019-42860-0.

190. Kleter, Cijs A., Ad A. C.M. Peijnenburg, and Henk J.M. Aarts. "Health Considerations Regarding Horizontal Transfer of Microbial Transgenes Present in Genetically Modified Crops", 2005. ncbi.nlm.nih.gov/pmc/articles/PMC1364539/.

191. Zhou, Wen. "The Patent Landscape of Genetically Modified Organisms." Science in the News, 11 Aug. 2015, sitn.hms.harvard.edu/flash/2015/the-patent-landscape-of-genetically-modified-organisms/.

192. Kubala, Jillian. "Is Canola Oil Healthy? All You Need to Kno ." Healthline.com , 7 Feb. 2019, healthline.com/nutrition/is-canola-oil-health

193. Leech , Joe. "11 Proven Benefits of Olive Oil ." Healthline.com , Sept. 2018, healthline.com/nutrition/11-proven-benefits-of-olive-oil.

194. "How Much Is Too Much?" SugarScience.UCSF.edu, 8 Dec. 2018, sugarscience.ucsf.edu/the-growing-concern-of-overconsumption.html#.XhptYy-ZPOR.

195. Lustig, Robert H. "Fructose: Metabolic, Hedonic, and Societal Parallels with Ethanol." Journal of the American Dietetic Association, U.S. National Library of Medicine, Sept. 2010, ncbi.nlm.nih.gov/pubmed/20800122.

196. "Laying Bare the Not-so-Sweet Tale of a Sugar and Its Role in the Spread of Cancer." ScienceDaily, ScienceDaily, 25 Apr. 2011, sciencedaily.com/releases/2011/04/110425120346.htm.

197. "Doctors Warn." Institute for Responsible Technology. responsibletechnology.org/doctors-warn/.

198. Rowe, Katherine S., and Kenneth J. Rowe. "Synthetic Food Coloring and Behavior: A Dose Response Effect in a Double-Blind, Placebo-Controlled, Repeated-Measures Study." *The Journal of Pediatrics*, Mosby, 20 Nov. 2007, sciencedirect.com/science/article/abs/pii/S0022347606801642.

199. Kavanagh, Kylie, Wylie, Ashley T, Tucker, Kelly, Hamp, Timothy J, Gharaibeh, Raad Z, Fodor, Anthony, Cullen, and John M. "Dietary Fructose Induces Endotoxemia and Hepatic Injury in Calorically Controlled Primates." OUP Academic. June 19, 2013. academic.oup.com/ajcn/article/98/2/349/4577187.

200. Janjua, Hafeez Ullah, Munir Akhtar, and Fayyaz Hussain. "Effects of Sugar, Salt and Distilled Water on White Blood Cells and Platelet Cells: A Review." Journal of Tumor. ghrnet.org/index.php/JT/article/view/1340/1795.

201. Sadowska, Joanna, and Magda Bruszkowska. "Comparing the Effects of Sucrose and High-Fructose Corn Syrup on Lipid Metabolism and the Risk of Cardiovascular Disease in Male Rats." Acta Scientiarum Polonorum. Technologia Alimentaria, U.S. National Library of Medicine, 2017, ncbi.nlm.nih.gov/pubmed/28703963.

202. Stanhope, Kimber L, et al. "Consuming Fructose-Sweetened, Not Glucose-Sweetened, Beverages Increases Visceral Adiposity and Lipids and Decreases Insulin Sensitivity in Overweight/Obese Humans." The Journal of Clinical Investigation, American Society for Clinical Investigation, May 2009, ncbi.nlm.nih.gov/pmc/articles/PMC2673878/.

203. Parker, Hilary. "A Sweet Problem: Princeton Researchers Find That High-Fructose Corn Syrup Prompts Considerably More Weight Gain." Princeton University, The Trustees of Princeton University, 2010, princeton.edu/news/2010/03/22/sweet-problem-princeton-researchers-find-high-fructose-corn-syrup-prompts.

204. Eteref-Oskouei, Tahereh, and Moslem Najafi. "Traditional and Modern Uses of Natural Honey in Human Diseases: A Review", July 16, 2013. ncbi.nlm.nih.gov/pmc/articles/PMC3758027/#B73.

205. Goyal, S K, et al. "Stevia (Stevia Rebaudiana) a Bio-Sweetener: a Review." *International Journal of Food Sciences and Nutrition*, U.S. National Library of Medicine, Feb. 2010, ncbi.nlm.nih.gov/pubmed/19961353.

206. Carrera-Lanestosa, Areli, et al. "Stevia Rebaudiana Bertoni: A Natural Alternative for Treating Diseases Associated with Metabolic Syndrome." *Mary Ann Liebert, Inc., Publishers*, 1 Oct. 2017, liebertpub.com/doi/abs/10.1089/jmf.2016.0171?journalCode=jmf.

207. Virgin, JJ. "Coconut Sugar: Healthier Sweetener or Another Pretty Name for Sugar?" HuffPost, HuffPost, 18 Oct. 2014, huffpost.com/entry/coconut-sugar-healthier-s_b_5669084.

208. Yamamoto, Tetsushi, et al. "Inhibitory Effect of Maple Syrup on the Cell Growth and Invasion of Human Colorectal Cancer Cells." Oncology Reports, D.A. Spandidos, Apr. 2015, ncbi.nlm.nih.gov/pmc/articles/PMC4358083/.

209. Li, Liya, and Navindra P Seeram. "Further Investigation into Maple Syrup Yields 3 New Lignans, a New Phenylpropanoid, and 26 Other Phytochemicals." Journal of Agricultural and Food Chemistry, U.S. National Library of Medicine, 27 July 2011, ncbi.nlm.nih.gov/pmc/articles/PMC3140541/.

210. Guri, Amir J, et al. "Abscisic Acid Synergizes with Rosiglitazone to Improve Glucose Tolerance and down-Modulate Macrophage Accumulation in Adipose Tissue: Possible Action of the CAMP/PKA/PPAR γ Axis." Clinical Nutrition (Edinburgh, Scotland), U.S. National Library of Medicine, Oct. 2010, ncbi.nlm.nih.gov/pmc/articles/PMC2888662/.

211. "How the Body Regulates Salt Levels." National Institutes of Health, U.S. Department of Health and Human Services, 12 May 2017, nih.gov/news-events/nih-research-matters/how-body-regulates-salt-levels.

212. "Salt and Sodium." The Nutrition Source, 16 Dec. 2019, hsph.harvard.edu/nutritionsource/salt-and-sodium/.[thekitchn.com/kosher-salt-where-it-comes-from-why-its-called-kosher-ingredient-intelligence-219665]

213. Ji-Su Kim, Hee-Jee Lee, Seung-Kyu Kim, and Hyun-Jung Kim. "Global Pattern of Microplastics (MPs) in Commercial Food-Grade Salts: Sea Salt as an Indicator of Seawater MP Pollution." *Environmental Science & Technology*. 2018 52 (21), 12819-12828 DOI: 10.1021/acs.est.8b04180

214. Pearson, Keith. "Is Pink Himalayan Salt Better Than Regular Salt?" Healthline.com , 16 May 2017, healthline.com/nutrition/pink-himalayan-salt.

215. Sciences, National Academies of, et al. "Human Health Effects of Genetically Engineered Crops." *Genetically Engineered Crops: Experiences and Prospects.*, U.S. National Library of Medicine, 17 May 2016, ncbi.nlm.nih.gov/books/NBK424534/.

216. Kurokawa, Y, et al. "Toxicity and Carcinogenicity of Potassium Bromate--a New Renal Carcinogen." *Environmental Health Perspectives*, U.S. National Library of Medicine, July 1990, ncbi.nlm.nih.gov/pmc/articles/PMC1567851/.

217. Szkudelski, T. (2001). The mechanism of alloxan and streptozotocin action in B cells of the rat pancreas. Physiological Research, 50(6), 537– 546.

218. Maldonado-Cervantes, Enrique, et al. "Amaranth Lunasin-like Peptide Internalizes into the Cell Nucleus and Inhibits Chemical Carcinogen-Induced Transformation of NIH-3T3 Cells." *Peptides*, U.S. National Library of Medicine, Sept. 2010, ncbi.nlm.nih.gov/pubmed/20599579.

219. Gong, Lingxiao, et al. "Intake of Tibetan Hull-Less Barley Is Associated with a Reduced Risk of Metabolic Related Syndrome in Rats Fed High-Fat-Sucrose Diets." Nutrients, MDPI, 21 Apr. 2014, ncbi.nlm.nih.gov/pmc/articles/PMC4011056/.

220. "A2 Milk Study: New Zealand Agricultural Research: AgResearch." *AgResearch* NZ, agresearch.co.nz/news/a2-milk-study/.

221. Abdelmonaim Azzouz, Beatriz Jurado-Sánchez, Badredine Souhail, and Evaristo Ballesteros. "Simultaneous Determination of 20 Pharmacologically Active Substances in Cow's Milk, Goat's Milk, and Human Breast Milk by Gas Chromatography—Mass Spectrometry." *Journal of Agricultural and Food Chemistry* 2011 59 (9), 5125-5132 DOI: 10.1021/jf200364w

222. "Fat Globules." *Fat Globules—an Overview | ScienceDirect Topics*, sciencedirect.com/topics/agricultural-and-biological-sciences/fat-globules.

223. Charles M. Benbrook, Donald R. Davis, Bradley J. Heins, Maged A. Latif, Carlo Leifert, Logan Peterman, Gillian Butler, Ole Faergeman, Silvia Abel-Caines, Marcin Baranski. "Enhancing the fatty acid profile of milk through forage-based rations, with nutrition modeling of diet outcomes." *Food Science & Nutrition*, 2018; DOI: 10.1002/fsn3.610

224. Andersen, Catherine J, et al. "Egg Consumption Modulates HDL Lipid Composition and Increases the Cholesterol-Accepting Capacity of Serum in Metabolic Syndrome." *Lipids*, U.S. National Library of Medicine, June 2013, ncbi.nlm.nih.gov/pubmed/23494579.

225. Park, Young W., and George F. W. Haenlein. *Milk and Dairy Products in Human Nutrition: Production, Composition and Health.* John Wiley & Sons, Ltd., 2013.

226. Harvard Health Publishing. "In Brief: Dietary Lutein and Zeaxanthin May Slow Macular Degeneration." *Harvard Health*, health.harvard.edu/newsletter_article/In_Brief_Dietary_lutein_and_zeaxanthin_may_slow_macular_degeneration.

227. "Tyrosine." *National Center for Biotechnology Information. PubChem Compound Database*, U.S. National Library of Medicine, pubchem.ncbi.nlm.nih.gov/compound/tyrosine.

228. Jenkins, Trisha A, et al. "Influence of Tryptophan and Serotonin on Mood and Cognition with a Possible Role of the Gut-Brain Axis." *Nutrients*, MDPI, 20 Jan. 2016, ncbi.nlm.nih.gov/pmc/articles/PMC4728667/.

229. "Tyrosine." *National Center for Biotechnology Information. PubChem Compound Database*, U.S. National Library of Medicine, pubchem.ncbi.nlm.nih.gov/compound/Tyrosine#section=Pharmacology-and-Biochemistry.

230. Karsten, H.D., et al. "Vitamins A, E and Fatty Acid Composition of the Eggs of Caged Hens and Pastured Hens: Renewable Agriculture and Food Systems." *Cambridge Core*, Cambridge University Press, 12 Jan. 2010, cambridge.org/core/journals/renewable-agriculture-and-food-systems/article/vitamins-a-e-and-fatty-acid-composition-of-the-eggs-of-caged-hens-and-pastured-hens/552BA04E5A9E3CD7E49E405B339ECA32.

231. Lot, Joanna. "Pasture-Ized Poultry." *Penn State University*, news.psu.edu/story/140750/2003/05/01/research/pasture-ized-poultry.

232. Nimalaratne, Chamila, et al. "Free Aromatic Amino Acids in Egg Yolk Show Antioxidant Properties." *Food Chemistry*, Elsevier, 1 May 2011, sciencedirect.com/science/article/pii/S0308814611006248.

233. Valenzuela, Alfonso, et al. "Cholesterol Oxidation: Health Hazard and the Role of Antioxidants in Prevention." *Biological Research*, U.S. National Library of Medicine, 2003, ncbi.nlm.nih.gov/pubmed/14631863.

234. Hunter, Aina. "Recalled Eggs List: Blame Factory Farms for Salmonella Outbreak?" *CBS News*, CBS Interactive, 23 Aug. 2010, cbsnews.com/news/recalled-eggs-list-blame-factory-farms-for-salmonella-outbreak/.

235. Karsten, H.D., et al. "Vitamins A, E and Fatty Acid Composition of the Eggs of Caged Hens and Pastured Hens: Renewable Agriculture and Food Systems." *Cambridge Core*, Cambridge University Press, 12 Jan. 2010, cambridge.org/core/journals/renewable-agriculture-and-food-systems/article/vitamins-a-e-and-fatty-acid-composition-of-the-eggs-of-caged-hens-and-pastured-hens/552BA04E5A9E3CD7E49E405B339ECA32.

236. Henriksen, Rie, et al. "Elevated Plasma Corticosterone Decreases Yolk Testosterone and Progesterone in Chickens: Linking Maternal Stress and Hormone-Mediated Maternal Effects." PLOS ONE, Public Library of Science, 2011, journals.plos.org/plosone/article?id=10.1371%2Fjournal.pone.0023824.

237. Medicine, C. F. (n.d.). Report on FDA Review of the Safety of Recombinant Bovine Somatotropin. Retrieved from fda.gov/animal-veterinary/product-safety-information/report-food-and-drug-administrations-review-safety-recombinant-bovine-somatotropin

238. "Record-High Antibiotic Sales for Meat and Poultry Production." The Pew Charitable Trusts, 2013, pewtrusts.org/en/research-and-analysis/articles/2013/02/06/recordhigh-antibiotic-sales-for-meat-and-poultry-production.

239. Landers, Timothy F, et al. "A Review of Antibiotic Use in Food Animals: Perspective, Policy, and Potential." *Public Health Reports (Washington, D.C. : 1974)*, Association of Schools of Public Health, 2012, ncbi.nlm.nih.gov/pmc/articles/PMC3234384/.

240. United States, Congress, Center for Disease Control. "Antibiotic Resistance Threats in the United States in 2013." CDC, 2013.

241. Hribar, Carrie. *Understanding Concentrated Animal Feeding Operations and Their Impact on Communities.* National Association of Local Boards of Health, 2010.

242. Melinda Moyer. "The Looming Threat of Factory-Farm Superbugs." *Scientific American.* 2016 Dec; 315, 6, 70-79. DOI:10.1038/scientificamerican1216-70.

243. Center for Disease Control, National Association of Local Boards of Health, and Carrie Hribar. "Understanding Concentrated Animal Feeding Operations and Their Impact on Communities." NALBOH, 2010.

244. Van Elswyk ME, McNeill SH. "Impact of grass/forage feeding versus grain finishing on beef nutrients and sensory quality: the U.S. experience." *Meat Science.* 2014 Jan;96(1):535-40. doi: 10.1016/j.meatsci.2013.08.010. Epub 2013 Aug 14.

245. Amy Lowman, Mary Anne McDonald, Steve Wing, Naeema Muhammad. "Land Application of Treated Sewage Sludge: Community Health and Environmental Justice." *Environmental Health Perspectives.* 2013 May 1. DOI: 10.1289/ehp.1205470.

246. Imhoff, D. (2010). *The CAFO reader: The tragedy of industrial animal factories.* Berkeley, CA: Watershed Media.

247. Grandin, T. (1980). The effect of stress on livestock and meat quality prior to and during slaughter. International Journal for the Study of Animal Problems, 1(5), 313-337.

248. Ferguson, Dwight D, et al. "Detection of Airborne Methicillin-Resistant Staphylococcus Aureus Inside and Downwind of a Swine Building, and in Animal Feed: Potential Occupational, Animal Health, and Environmental Implications." *Journal of Agromedicine*, U.S. National Library of Medicine, 2016, ncbi.nlm.nih.gov/pubmed/26808288.

249. Casey, Joan A, et al. "High-Density Livestock Operations, Crop Field Application of Manure, and Risk of Community-Associated Methicillin-Resistant Staphylococcus Aureus Infection in Pennsylvania." *JAMA Internal Medicine*, U.S. National Library of Medicine, 25 Nov. 2013, ncbi.nlm.nih.gov/pubmed/24043228.

250. Descalzo, A M, et al. "Antioxidant Status and Odour Profile in Fresh Beef from Pasture or Grain-Fed Cattle." *Meat Science*, U.S. National Library of Medicine, Feb. 2007, ncbi.nlm.nih.gov/pubmed/22063662.

251. McAfee, A J, et al. "Red Meat from Animals Offered a Grass Diet Increases Plasma and Platelet n-3 PUFA in Healthy Consumers." *The British Journal of Nutrition*, U.S. National Library of Medicine, Jan. 2011, ncbi.nlm.nih.gov/pubmed/20807460.

252. Bhattacharya, A., Banu, J., Rahman, M., et al. Biological effects of conjugated linoleic acid in health and disease. J. Nutr. Biochem. 17: 789-810, 2006.

253. Parodi, P W. "Conjugated Linoleic Acid and Other Anticarcinogenic Agents of Bovine Milk Fat." *Journal of Dairy Science*, U.S. National Library of Medicine, June 1999, ncbi.nlm.nih.gov/pubmed/10386321.

254. Tianxi Yang, Jeffery Doherty, Bin Zhao, Amanda J. Kinchla, John M. Clark, Lili He. "Effectiveness of Commercial and Homemade Washing Agents in Removing Pesticide Residues on and in Apples." *Journal of Agricultural and Food Chemistry.* 2017 65 (44), 9744-9752 DOI: 10.1021/acs.jafc.7b03118

255. Environmental Working Group. "EWG's 2019 Shopper's Guide to Pesticides in Produce™." *EWG's 2019 Shopper's Guide to Pesticides in Produce | Summary*, ewg.org/foodnews/summary.php.

256. Kapadia GJ, Azuine MA, Rao GS, Arai T, Iida A, Tokuda H. "Cytotoxic effect of the red beetroot (Beta vulgaris L.) extract compared to doxorubicin (Adriamycin) in the human prostate (PC-3) and breast (MCF-7) cancer cell lines." *Anticancer Agents Med Chem.* 2011 Mar;11(3):280-4.

257. Webb, Andrew J, et al. "Acute Blood Pressure Lowering, Vasoprotective, and Antiplatelet Properties of Dietary Nitrate via Bioconversion to Nitrite." *Hypertension (Dallas, Tex. : 1979)*, U.S. National Library of Medicine, Mar. 2008, ncbi.nlm.nih.gov/pubmed/18250365.

258. Asgary, S, et al. "Improvement of Hypertension, Endothelial Function and Systemic Inflammation Following Short-Term Supplementation with Red Beet (Beta Vulgaris L.) Juice: a Randomized Crossover Pilot Study." *Journal of Human Hypertension*, U.S. National Library of Medicine, Oct. 2016, ncbi.nlm.nih.gov/pubmed/27278926.

259. Clifford, Tom, et al. "The Potential Benefits of Red Beetroot Supplementation in Health and Disease." *Nutrients*, MDPI, 14 Apr. 2015, ncbi.nlm.nih.gov/pmc/articles/PMC4425174/.

260. "Folic Acid: Why You Need It When Getting Pregnant: ConceiveEasy." *ConceiveEasy.com*, 29 Jan. 2019, conceiveeasy.com/get-pregnant/folic-acid-why-you-need-it-when-getting-pregnant/.

261. Arsalan. "Effect of Yeast on Different Types of Sugar to Produce CO2." *Academic Master*, 30 Apr. 2019, academic-master.com/effect-of-yeast-on-different-types-os-sugar-to-produce-co2/.

262. Klewicka, Elżbieta, et al. "Effects of Lactofermented Beetroot Juice Alone or with N-Nitroso-N-Methylurea on Selected Metabolic Parameters, Composition of the Microbiota Adhering to the Gut Epithelium and Antioxidant Status of Rats." *Nutrients*, MDPI, 16 July 2015, ncbi.nlm.nih.gov/pmc/articles/PMC4517037/.

263. Edison Institute of Nutrition. "The Dangers of Aggressive Detoxing." *Edison Institute of Nutrition*, 19 Feb. 2020, edisoninst.com/why-your-detox-is-making-you-sick-the-dangers-of-aggressive-detoxing/.

264. "Children Exposed Daily to Personal Care Products With Chemicals Not Found Safe For Kids." *EWG*, ewg.org/news/news-releases/2007/11/01/children-exposed-daily-personal-care-products-chemicals-not-found-safe.

265. Cosmetics Ingredient Review (CIR) (2003). 2003 CIR Compendium, containing abstracts, discussions, and conclusions of CIR cosmetic ingredient safety assessments. Washington DC.

266. "Bronopol." *National Center for Biotechnology Information. PubChem Compound Database*, U.S. National Library of Medicine, pubchem.ncbi.nlm.nih.gov/compound/bronopol#section=GHS-Classification.

267. "1,3-Bis(Hydroxymethyl)-5,5-Dimethylimidazolidine-2,4-Dione." *National Center for Biotechnology Information. PubChem Compound Database*, U.S. National Library of Medicine, pubchem.ncbi.nlm.nih.gov/compound/DMDM-Hydantoin#section=Acute-Effects.

268. Park, Chan Jin, et al. "Sanitary Pads and Diapers Contain Higher Phthalate Contents than Those in Common Commercial Plastic Products." *Reproductive Toxicology*, Pergamon, 16 Jan. 2019, sciencedirect.com/science/article/pii/S0890623818302259?via%3Dihub.

269. "Phthalates." *Phthalates—an Overview | ScienceDirect Topics*, sciencedirect.com/topics/earth-and-planetary-sciences/phthalates.

270. "Acute Respiratory Effects of Diaper Emissions." *Taylor & Francis*, tandfonline.com/doi/abs/10.1080/00039899909602500.

271. Anderson, R C, and J H Anderson. "Acute Respiratory Effects of Diaper Emissions." *Archives of Environmental Health*, U.S. National Library of Medicine, 1999, ncbi.nlm.nih.gov/pubmed/10501153.

272. "Nondurable Goods: Product-Specific Data." *United States Environmental Protection Agency*. epa.gov/facts-and-figures-about-materials-waste-and-recycling/nondurable-goods-product-specific-data#DisposableDiapers

273. "Soy Infant Formula." *National Institute of Environmental Health Sciences*, U.S. Department of Health and Human Services, niehs.nih.gov/health/topics/agents/sya-soy-formula/index.cfm.

274. Tobacman, J. K. (2001). Review of Harmful Gastrointestinal Effects of Carrageenan in Animal Experiments. *Environmental Health Perspectives*, 109(10), 983. doi:10.2307/3454951

275. Vallaeys, Charlotte. "Replacing Mother--Imitating Human Breast Milk in the Laboratory." *Cornucopia Institute*, Jan. 2008, cornucopia.org/DHA/DHA_FullReport.pdf.

276. Ewg. "EWG's Food Scores Just Took the Work out of Grocery Shopping for Me!" *EWG*, ewg.org/foodscores/products/070074647883-SimilacOptigroMilkBasedPowder.

277. Jackson, Brian P et al. "Arsenic, organic foods, and brown rice syrup." *Environmental health perspectives* vol. 120,5 (2012): 623-6. doi:10.1289/ehp.1104619

278. Breastfeeding, Section On. "Breastfeeding and the Use of Human Milk." *American Academy of Pediatrics*, American Academy of Pediatrics, 1 Mar. 2012, pediatrics.aappublications.org/content/129/3/e827.

279. "Benefits of Breastfeeding." *AAP.org*, aap.org/en-us/advocacy-and-policy/aap-health-initiatives/Breastfeeding/Pages/Benefits-of-Breastfeeding.aspx.

280. Pal, Sanghamitra, et al. "Bisphenol S Impairs Blood Functions and Induces Cardiovascular Risks in Rats." *Toxicology Reports*, Elsevier, 20 Oct. 2017, sciencedirect.com/science/article/pii/S2214750017300732.

281. Chun Z. Yang, Stuart I. Yaniger, V. Craig Jordan, Daniel J. Klein, George D. Bittner. "Most Plastic Products Release Estrogenic Chemicals: A Potential Health Problem That Can Be Solved." *Environmental Health Perspectives*. 2011 July 1. doi: 10.1289/ehp.1003220

282. Brandon E. Boor, Helena Järnström, Atila Novoselac, Ying Xu. "Infant Exposure to Emissions of Volatile Organic Compounds from Crib Mattresses." *Environmental Science & Technology*. 2014 48 (6), 3541-3549. DOI: 10.1021/es405625q

283. Brandon E. Boor, Yirui Liang, Neil E. Crain, Helena Järnström, Atila Novoselac, Ying Xu. "Identification of Phthalate and Alternative Plasticizers, Flame Retardants, and Unreacted Isocyanates in Infant Crib Mattress Covers and Foam." *Environmental Science & Technology Letters*. 2015 2 (4), 89-94. DOI: 10.1021/acs.estlett.5b00039

284. Tappin, David, et al. "Used Infant Mattresses and Sudden Infant Death Syndrome in Scotland: Case-Control Study." *The BMJ*, British Medical Journal Publishing Group, 2 Nov. 2002, bmj.com/content/325/7371/1007.1/rapid-responses.

285. "Exposure to Pet and Pest Allergens during Infancy Linked to Reduced Asthma Risk." National Institutes of Health, U.S. Department of Health and Human Services, 2 Oct. 2017, nih.gov/news-events/news-releases/exposure-pet-pest-allergens-during-infancy-linked-reduced-asthma-risk.

286. "About Pets & People." *Centers for Disease Control and Prevention.* cdc.gov/healthypets/health-benefits/

287. "Pet Owners—Disease Information." (2018, July 30). National Cancer Institute ccr.cancer.gov/Comparative-Oncology-Program/pet-owners/disease-info

288. Pokorny, Kym. "Flame Retardant May Cause Hyperthyroidism in Cats." *Phys.org*, Phys.org, 13 Aug. 2019, phys.org/news/2019-08-flame-retardant-hyperthyroidism-cats.html.

289. Edie Lau. "Lawsuits proliferate against makers of topical flea and tick products." *Vin News Service.* 2010 Mar 26. news.vin.com/doc/?id=4442412

290. "Treating Bacterial Infections in Dogs with Betadine Solution." *VetInfo*, vetinfo.com/treating-bacterial-infections-in-dogs-with-betadine-solution.html.

291. Riva, Gretel Torres de la, et al. "Neutering Dogs: Effects on Joint Disorders and Cancers in Golden Retrievers." *PLOS ONE*, Public Library of Science, journals.plos.org/plosone/article?id=10.1371%2Fjournal.pone.0055937.

292. Hofve, Dr. Jean. "Inflammatory Bowel Disease (IBD) in Dogs & Cats." *Only Natural Pet*, Dec. 2019, onlynaturalpet.com/blogs/holistic-healthcare-library/inflammatory-bowel-disease.

293. "Is It Okay To Give My Dog A Bone? Which Bones Are Safe For Dogs?" *Dogtime*, 8 Nov. 2018, dogtime.com/dog-health/dog-food-dog-nutrition/52539-ok-give-dog-bone-bones-safe-dogs.

294. Lanigan RS. "Final report on the safety assessment of Sodium Metaphosphate, Sodium Trimetaphosphate, and Sodium Hexametaphosphate." *Int J Toxicol.* 2001;20 Suppl 3:75-89.

295. "Bentonite Material Safety Data Sheet." *ECCA Holdings.* 2005 Jan 14. capebentonite.co.za/downloads/BENTONITE%20MATERIAL%20SAFETY%20DATA%20SHEET.pdf

296. "Department of Animal Science—Plants Poisonous to Livestock." *Cornell University Department of Animal Science*, poisonousplants.ansci.cornell.edu/toxicagents/aflatoxin/aflatoxin.html.

297. Kosicek, Marko, and Silva Hecimovic. "Phospholipids and Alzheimer's Disease: Alterations, Mechanisms and Potential Biomarkers." *International Journal of Molecular Sciences*, MDPI, 10 Jan. 2013, ncbi.nlm.nih.gov/pmc/articles/PMC3565322/.

298. Cherry, Kendra. "The Color Psychology of Green ." *Verywell Mind*, Verywell Mind, 24 Sept. 2019, verywellmind.com/color-psychology-green-2795817.

299. "Senior Research Scientist at MIT Shows How Massive Spike in Disease Is Correlated with Glyphosate in Roundup's Weedkiller." *Weed Killer Crisis*, 22 Aug. 2019, weedkillercrisis.com/topics/glyphosate-report-2019/.

300. "Pesticide Exposure in Children." *Council On Environmental Health* Pediatrics Dec 2012, 130 (6) e1757-e1763; DOI: 10.1542/peds.2012-2757

301. Cowles, Richard S., and Brian D. Eitzer. "Residues of Neonicotinoid Insecticides in Pollen and Nectar from Model Plants." *Journal of Environmental Horticulture*, Mar. 2017, hrijournal.org/doi/full/10.24266/0738-2898-35.1.24.

302. Gottlieb, Barbara, et al. "Coal Ash: The Toxic Threat to Our Health and Environment." *Physicians for Social Responsibility and EarthJustice*, Sept. 2010, psr.org/wp-content/uploads/2018/05/coal-ash.pdf.

303. "Inventory and Emission Factors of Creosote, Polycyclic Aromatic Hydrocarbons (PAH), and Phenols from Railroad Ties Treated with Creosote." *Environmental Science & Technology*, pubs.acs.org/doi/abs/10.1021/es000103h.

304. "Toxic Substances Portal—Creosote." *Centers for Disease Control and Prevention*, Centers for Disease Control and Prevention, atsdr.cdc.gov/phs/phs.asp?id=64&tid=18.

305. Tarazona, Jose V et al. "Glyphosate toxicity and carcinogenicity: a review of the scientific basis of the European Union assessment and its differences with IARC." *Archives of toxicology* vol. 91,8 (2017): 2723-2743. doi:10.1007/s00204-017-1962-5

306. "Community and Environment." *Washington State Department of Health*, doh.wa.gov/CommunityandEnvironment/AirQuality/IndoorAir/Fiberglass.

307. "Potential Chemical Exposures From Spray Polyurethane Foam." *EPA*, Environmental Protection Agency, 14 May 2019, epa.gov/saferchoice/potential-chemical-exposures-spray-polyurethane-foam.

308. Corscadden, K.W., et al. "Sheep's Wool Insulation: A Sustainable Alternative Use for a Renewable Resource?" *Resources, Conservation and Recycling*, Elsevier, 23 Feb. 2014, sciencedirect.com/science/article/pii/S0921344914000202.

309. "Natural Wool Insulation Full Benefits." *NATURAL WOOL INSULATION*, naturalwoolinsulation.com/natural-wool-insulation-full-benefits/.

310. "Basic Radon Factsheet." *United States Environmental Protection Agency*, July 2016, epa.gov/sites/production/files/2016-08/documents/july_2016_radon_factsheet.pdf.

311. Weinhold, Bob. "A spreading concern: inhalational health effects of mold." *Environmental health perspectives* vol. 115,6 (2007): A300-5. doi:10.1289/ehp.115-a300